CENTRAL NERVOUS SYSTEM
CLINICAL ALGORITHMS

CENTRAL NERVOUS SYSTEM
CLINICAL ALGORITHMS

Published by the British Medical Journal
Tavistock Square, London WC1H 9JR

First Edition 1989

ISBN 0-7279-0256-3

Printed in Great Britain by Cambridge University Press
Typesetting by Bedford Typesetters Ltd, Bedford

Contents

MANAGEMENT OF EPILEPSY

A K SCOTT

The patient with epilepsy usually presents with a history of one or more attacks. If epilepsy is diagnosed the type of disorder should be established from the clinical features and electroencephalographic changes. A complex internationally agreed classification of epileptic seizures has been produced; a simplified version is shown in the table, together with suitable anticonvulsant treatment.

The order of decisions about management is shown in the algorithm.

(1) *Is it an epileptic attack?* This is a clinical diagnosis and is helped by an informed eye witness account of the episode as well as the presence of characteristics such as an aura, tonic-clonic movements, incontinence, tongue biting, and the nature of recovery after the episode. By definition a patient should not be labelled "epileptic" until two attacks have occurred.

(2) *Does an examination of the central nervous system yield normal results?* Any abnormality requires full investigation. Additional investigations to those shown are occasionally indicated. These include lumbar puncture and cerebral angiograms.

(3) *How old is the patient?* Underlying causes become more common in epilepsy presenting for the first time in patients over the age of 25. More complete investigation should be considered in patients over this age.

(4) *Are the investigation results helpful?* The underlying causative lesion may be removed in some patients—for example, by excision of a meningioma. All patients with an underlying cause should also be treated with an anticonvulsant.

(5) *How many fits have occurred?* An isolated fit does not require treatment. The occurrence of two or more fits requires anticonvulsant therapy, though the risks of treatment must be balanced against those of the disease. Consideration of the legal requirements for possessing a driving licence—for example, freedom from fits while awake for at least two years—may favour treatment in patients with very infrequent seizures.

(6) *Which anticonvulsant?* The choice of drug depends on the pattern and type of seizure (see table). Individual factors may alter the order of choice. For example, young women may prefer carbamazepine or sodium valproate to avoid the cosmetic effects of phenytoin. If a future pregnancy is a possibility, carbamazepine is preferable to phenytoin or sodium valproate as it seems to cause less fetal abnormality.

Unless the fits are frequent and severe, the patient may be managed as an outpatient. The initial dose of the selected drug is given—for example, phenytoin 200-300 mg/day. The serum concentration of the drug is measured after it has reached steady state (4×drug half life)—usually one to two weeks. The relation of serum drug concentration to control of seizures is well established for phenytoin but less so for other drugs. Total drug (bound and free) concentrations are measured in most laboratories, whereas the free drug is considered to be active. The relative proportion of free drug may be increased in the presence of other drugs owing to displacement from plasma proteins—for example, sodium valproate displaces phenytoin—or if there is hypoalbuminaemia. In such circumstances a total drug concentration below the therapeutic range may be enough to produce an effective free drug concentration.

Doses should be altered in the light of control of fits and toxicity. The serum drug concentration is a secondary consideration if the patient is well. If fits are not controlled the dose of the drug of first choice should be increased to achieve a serum concentration at the upper limit of the therapeutic range before another drug is added. A second drug may then be added if there has been some reduction in the frequency of fits. If there has been no improvement a second drug should be added while the first is withdrawn over several days. A third drug is rarely needed. A second drug should also be substituted if the first has produced side effects not related to dose; then the first drug may have to be stopped abruptly and a loading dose of the substitute drug given over 24 hours to avoid withdrawal fits.

There are particular problems with phenytoin treatment because increasing the dose produces a disproportionate rise in the serum phenytoin concentration owing to the limited capacity of the enzymes concerned in its metabolism.

The patient's failure to take drugs must always be considered if serum concentrations are low in relation to the dose given.

The occurrence of side effects may necessitate a reduction in dosage or a change of drug.

Once fits are controlled the patient requires only infrequent monitoring—once a year or less.

Simplified classification of epileptic seizures with anticonvulsant of choice

Seizure type	1st Choice	2nd Choice
Generalised seizures		
Absence seizures:		
typical (petit mal)	Sodium valproate	Ethosuximide
atypical	Sodium valproate	Clonazepam
Myoclonic seizures	Sodium valproate	Clonazepam
Tonic-clonic seizures (grand mal)	Phenytoin, carbamazepine	Sodium valproate
Partial seizures		
Simple/complex	Carbamazepine	Phenytoin
(temporal lobe, Jacksonian, psychomotor seizures)		
Partial becoming generalised	Carbamazepine	Phenytoin

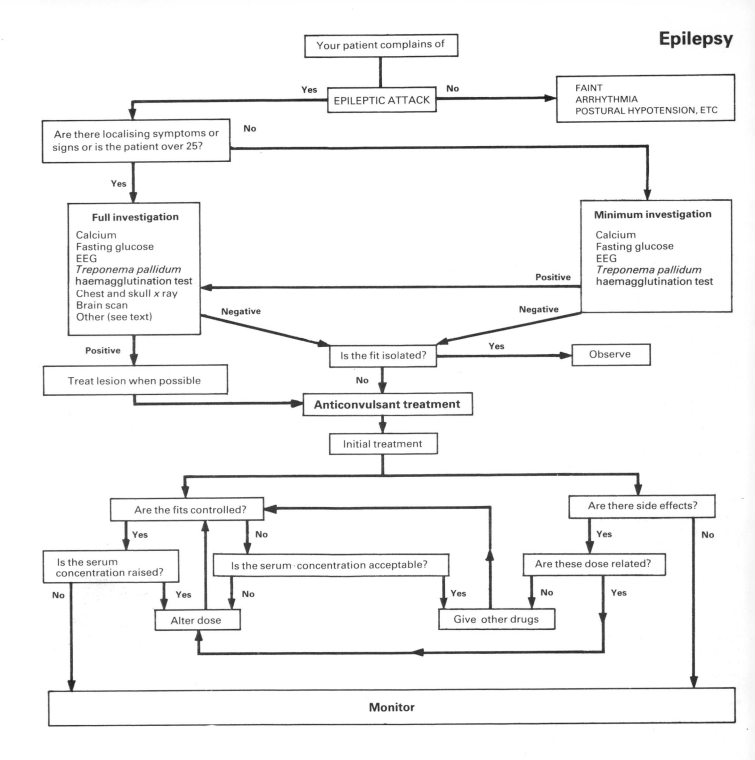

Points to note

First, the electroencephalogram is diagnostic of epilepsy in less than 50% of patients. It may be normal between attacks. Secondly, when phenytoin is used the dose must be increased in small increments (25 or 50 mg) above a dose of 300 mg daily, or a nomogram may be used. Thirdly, single drug therapy will control fits in most patients, provided adequate serum concentrations are achieved. For example, phenytoin or carbamazepine will bring about control in at least 80% of patients with grand mal attacks.

Finally, the patient or parents should be warned about important side effects. For example, dizziness, ataxia, visual disturbance, or excessive tiredness may suggest excessive dosage of phenytoin or carbamazepine; rash may occur with most drugs; sore throat may point to neutropenia (rare); hair loss may ocur with valproate. The need for good dental hygiene to reduce gingival hyperplasia should be explained for patients treated with phenytoin. On the return visit these side effects should be considered and the patient examined. Liver function tests should be performed every two months for six months after starting valproate. Enzyme inducing drugs (phenytoin, carbamazepine, phenobarbitone) may raise serum γ-glutamyltranspeptidase and alkaline phosphatase activities. This does not imply liver disease (the serum bilirubin concentration is lowered). Long term treatment with enzyme inducing drugs may cause low red blood cell folate and serum calcium concentrations and occasionally megalobastic anaemia and osteomalacia.

TREMOR

J E C HERN

Tremor is unwanted movement in which rhythmical oscillations occur. This rhythmical character distinguishes tremor from other involuntary movements. When formally analysed most tremors contain a range of frequencies, varying from 1–2 Hz up to 12 Hz or higher. This article considers certain common tremors that interfere with the use of the arms and legs. Clonus, a tremor that is seen most clearly when a muscle is passively stretched, is not considered, and rarer forms of tremor have been described elsewhere.[1]

In clinical practice tremors are usually identified by simple clinical examination, without the use of apparatus for recording and analysing their frequencies. The algorithm suggests a scheme for such identification, requiring observation of the tremor at rest, on sustained posture, and on active use of the limb. Postural tremor is usually shown when the patient holds out his arms with the fingers abducted or holds his finger to his nose with the arm abducted at the shoulder. Tremor on active use can be shown if he carries out an everyday task such as picking up and drinking from a glass. On the examination couch tremor is usually shown by the finger to nose or heel to shin tests.

Whatever its cause, tremor is commonly made worse by anxiety. This may lead patients, relatives, and even doctors wrongly to ascribe the tremor to emotional causes. Conversely, successful efforts to reduce anxiety, through reassurance, alcohol, or other sedative drugs, are likely to reduce the severity of tremor regardless of its cause.

Individual tremors and their treatments

Parkinsonian tremor is typically evident when the affected limb is not in use—for example, in the leg when a patient is sitting or lying and in the arm when he lets his arm hang by his side. It is less evident on active use but may persist during sustained posture. At the start tremor may affect one limb or one side alone but in severe cases may be generalised. Frequency is commonly around 4–5 Hz. The diagnosis can usually be confirmed by the presence of other parkinsonian features, especially bradykinesia and the characteristic stooped posture. If the tremor does not appreciably interfere with the use of the limb treatment with drugs may not be necessary. The patient may feel some social embarrassment, but drugs will rarely reduce the tremor enough to prevent this. If important bradykinesia is also present preparations containing levodopa, such as Madopar or Sinemet, are likely to be given but are usually of less benefit to tremor than to bradykinesia. Anticholinergic drugs, such as benzhexol, are worth using for tremor and can readily be combined with levodopa. If tremor is severe and responds inadequately to drugs stereotactic surgery should be considered. Anticholinergic drugs may also help if the parkinsonian tremor is drug induced, but the possibility of reducing or replacing the provoking drug should be considered. Prochlorperazine (Stemetil) is an example of a phenothiazine that can cause parkinsonism. This is commonly forgotten when the drug is used for nausea or vomiting.

Increased physiological tremor[2]—A tremor of the hands of low amplitude is present in all normal subjects. Frequency is in the range 6–12 Hz, tending to fall with increasing age.[3] Increased amplitude can be readily seen if the hands are held out with the fingers abducted. This type of postural tremor is of smaller amplitude than others; hence the distinction between fine and coarse in the algorithm. When possible the underlying cause should be treated. If immediate symptomatic suppression is needed β blockers, such as propranolol, are usually effective.

Drug related tremor[1]—A tremor comparable to essential tremor occurs in 40% of patients treated with lithium for manic depressive states. A similar tremor is sometimes seen with other drugs, including imipramine and amitriptyline. It is treated by reducing the dose or changing the drug.

Asterixis, or "flapping" tremor, is seen when the hands are outstretched: the posture is broken by a brief movement of flexion at wrist and fingers and is as quickly restored. Other forms of postural tremor may occur in the same circumstances.[4] Although classically associated with hepatic disease, asterixis may be seen in several metabolic disturbances, including renal and respiratory failure.[5] Treatment is of the underlying metabolic cause.

Essential tremor is a pure postural tremor of a frequency similar to that of physiological tremor[2] but of much greater amplitude. It may not develop until late in life (senile tremor) and tends to increase in severity with time. It is commonly hereditary, being inherited as an autosomal dominant condition, but many apparently sporadic cases are also seen. A striking feature, at times of some diagnostic help, is the extent to which it may improve with modest quantities of alcohol. Patients with essential tremor are often misdiagnosed as having Parkinson's disease. This may lead to distress and to treatment with antiparkinsonian drugs, to the disappointment of patient and doctor. If the criteria given in the algorithm are followed this error should seldom occur. Treatment is difficult. Alcohol or other sedation may suppress the tremor in the short term but is probably best reserved for occasions of particular social pressure as continued use may lead to addiction. Primidone has been reported to be helpful,[6] but my experience has not been encouraging. Propranolol or other β blocker may be helpful in some patients.

Cerebellar action and intention tremors—The classic intention tremor is most clearly seen towards the end of the movements in the finger to nose test. In some patients cerebellar tremors may be more prominent during the middle ranges of the movement and may also persist during sustained posture.[4 5] These tremors occur, for example, with lesions of the cerebellar pathways in multiple sclerosis, with brain stem vascular lesions, and with tumours. Symptomatic treatment is unsatisfactory. Choline has produced conflicting results.[5] If possible the underlying cause should be treated.

References

[1] Rondot P, Jedynak CP, Ferrey G. Pathological tremors: nosological correlates. In: Desmedt JE, ed. *Progress in clinical neurophysiology*. Vol 5. Basel: Karger, 1978: 95–113.

[2] Marsden CD. The mechanisms of physiological tremor and their significance for pathological tremors. In: Desmedt JE, ed. *Progress in clinical neurophysiology*. Vol 5. Basel: Karger, 1978: 1–16.

[3] Marshall J. The effect of ageing upon physiological tremor. *J Neurol Neurosurg Psychiatry* 1961;24:14–7.

[4] Marshall J. Tremor in Vinken and Bruyn. *Handbook of clinical neurology*. Vol 6. Amsterdam: North-Holland, 1968:809–25.

[5] Findlay LJ, Gresty MA. Tremor. *Br J Hosp Med* 1981;26:16–32.

[6] O'Brien MD, Upton AR, Toseland PA. Benign familial tremor treated with primidone. *Br Med J* 1981;282:178–80.

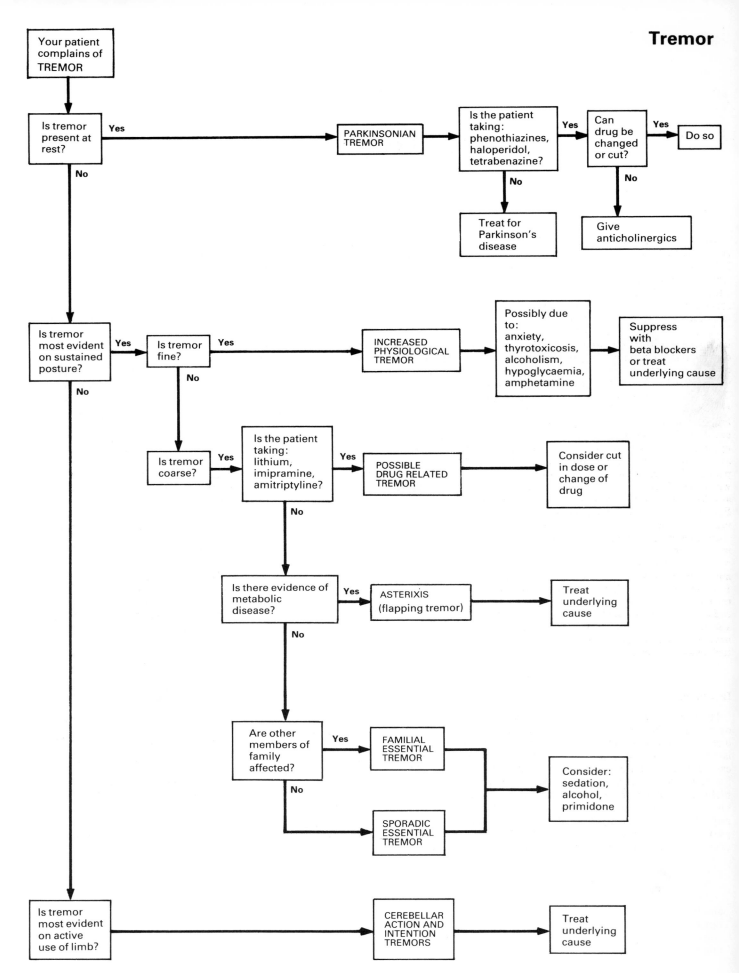

SYNCOPE

ANTHONY D ORMEROD

Transient loss of consciousness may be due to syncope, epilepsy, cardiac arrhythmia, and, rarely, transient cerebral ischaemic attack. It is important not to attribute syncope to cerebrovascular disease when the true cause is a transient disturbance of cardiac rhythm which is amenable to therapy. The differences between epilepsy and syncope will usually be apparent from a carefully taken history and whenever possible from an eye witness account.

Syncope is sudden, brief loss of consciousness due to transient impairment of cerebral circulation, from whatever cause, usually occurring in the absence of organic brain disease or cerebrovascular disease. Typically the onset is sudden or develops over a few seconds with blurred vision, dizziness, cold extremities, and perspiration. These features may give enough warning for the sufferer to take evasive action such as sitting down; otherwise the patient becomes limp and sinks to the ground with sighing respirations, pallor, and sweating. If venous return is impaired by the patient being propped up, or if the attack is prolonged, muscle twitching and convulsions may occur. These are rare but may confuse the diagnosis. The patient with syncope may complain of funny spells or dizzy turns in which consciousness is altered but not lost. The setting in which the attack occurs may help to distinguish the simple faint from epilepsy. For example, faints commonly occur in warm weather, when standing for prolonged periods, or after venepuncture.

In epilepsy the patient is usually rigid rather than limp; the onset is more abrupt, with injury and sometimes incontinence; and recovery is slow with confusion and drowsiness. The presence of an aura or perceptive or motor disturbances may all point to epilepsy. Fits and faints can both be precipitated by emotion and can both be related to the menstrual cycle. In transient ischaemic attacks consciousness is not usually lost unless the basilar artery territory is affected or there is global ischaemia. These patients will usually have focal neurological symptoms such as vertigo, visual disturbances, or ataxia.

Investigations

History and examination are the most important factors in determining the cause of syncope. In those patients for whom a diagnosis is not apparent on initial assessment further investigation is often fruitless and needs to be carefully directed to ensure the exclusion of sinister causes.[1] Most patients have a good prognosis but those over 70 years and those with a cardiac cause are at a much higher risk of death or major morbidity.[2] In the young patient with a history suggestive of a simple faint no further investigation is required. In the older patient this diagnosis should be made with great caution as cardiac dysrhythmia is more likely. In the elderly drugs are frequently to blame and many factors may operate together.

In all but the common faint an electrocardiograph is mandatory. During the electrocardiogram carotid sinus massage will reveal carotid sinus hypersensitivity and may uncover an underlying conduction defect. This is best done with the patient lying at 45° for five seconds only, on one side only, and with facilities for resuscitation at hand.[3] A full blood count may help to exclude anaemia or blood loss; serum electrolyte concentrations may indicate dehydration, Addison's disease, or hypocalcaemic and uraemic causes of convulsions; chest radiographs might show evidence of intrinsic cardiac disease or pulmonary embolism.

In a review of 121 patients with syncope in whom the diagnosis was undetermined by initial assessment a definitive cause was found in only 13.[4] By far the single most useful test was 24 hour continuous ambulatory electrocardiography, although careful interpretation is required to decide whether the abnormalities found explain the patient's symptoms. In the population studied computed tomography, radionuclide scanning, skull radiography, lumbar puncture, and glucose tolerance tests did not aid the diagnosis in any of the patients. Echocardiography, cardiac catheterisation, and electrophysiological studies were of intermediate value. Recent evidence suggests that electrophysiological studies are the most sensitive indicator of cardiac arrhythmia. In 149 patients with negative results from exhaustive investigations, including 24 hour continuous ambulatory electrocardiographic monitoring, 63% showed positive results, and with appropriate therapy 87% of these patients became free of symptoms[5]; the technique reveals a high incidence of unsuspected paroxysmal ventricular tachycardia not detected by non-invasive methods. It is, however, more expensive and invasive than 24 hour electrocardiographic monitoring and requires a skilled operator. There may be a place for empirical permanent pacing of patients with a suspected conduction abnormality not confirmed by investigation.[6]

References

[1] Critchley EMR, Wright JS. Evaluation of syncope. *Br Med J* 1983;**286**:500-1.
[2] Day SC, Cook EF, Funkenstein H, Goldman L. Evaluation and outcome of emergency room patients with transient loss of consciousness. *Am J Med* 1982;**73**:15-23.
[3] Davies AB, Stephens MR, Davies AG. Carotid sinus hypersensitivity in patients presenting with syncope. *Br Heart J* 1979;**42**:583-6.
[4] Kapoor WN, Karpf M, Maher Y, Miller RA, Levey GS. Syncope of unknown origin. The need for a more cost-effective approach to its diagnostic evaluation. *JAMA* 1982;**247**:2687-91.
[5] Camm AJ, Levy AM. Evaluation of syncope. *Br Med J* 1983;**286**:895.
[6] Gulamhusein S, Naccarelli GV, Ko PT, *et al*. Value and limitations of clinical electrophysiologic study in assessment of patients with unexplained syncope. *Am J Med* 1982;**73**:700-5.

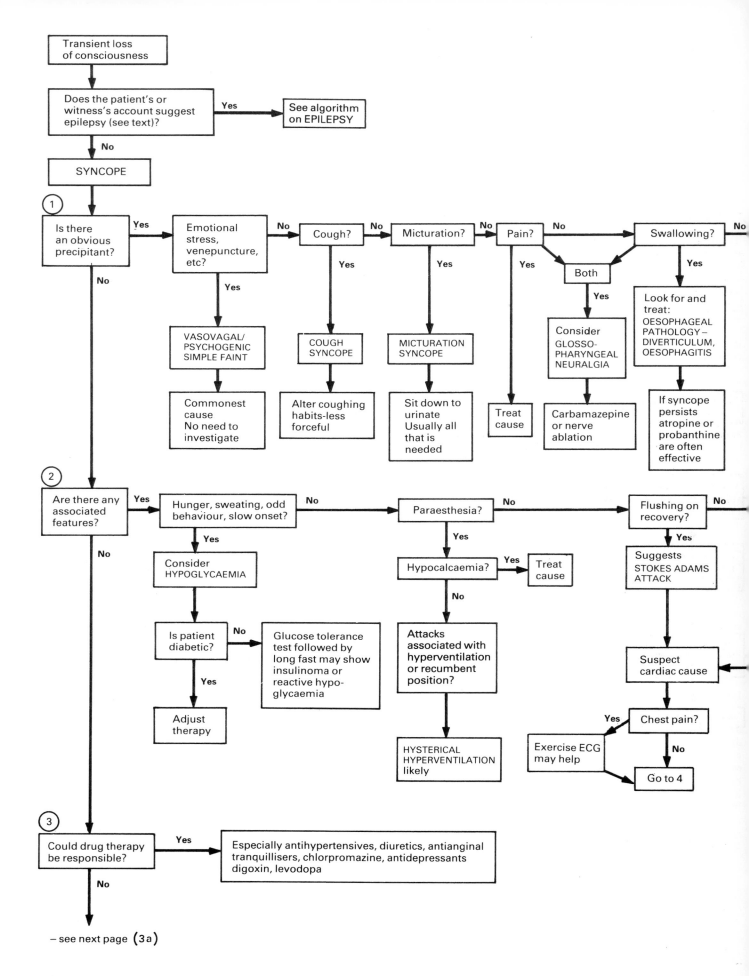

Transient loss of consciousness

Does the patient's or witness's account suggest epilepsy (see text)? — **Yes** → See algorithm on EPILEPSY

No

SYNCOPE

① Is there an obvious precipitant? — **Yes** → Emotional stress, venepuncture, etc?

— **No** → Cough? — **No** → Micturition? — **No** → Pain? — **No** → Swallowing? — **No**

Emotional stress, venepuncture, etc? — **Yes** → VASOVAGAL/ PSYCHOGENIC SIMPLE FAINT → Commonest cause No need to investigate

Cough? — **Yes** → COUGH SYNCOPE → Alter coughing habits-less forceful

Micturition? — **Yes** → MICTURITION SYNCOPE → Sit down to urinate Usually all that is needed

Pain? — **Yes** → Treat cause

Both — **Yes** → Consider GLOSSO-PHARYNGEAL NEURALGIA → Carbamazepine or nerve ablation

Swallowing? — **Yes** → Look for and treat: OESOPHAGEAL PATHOLOGY – DIVERTICULUM, OESOPHAGITIS → If syncope persists atropine or probanthine are often effective

No (from obvious precipitant)

② Are there any associated features? — **Yes** → Hunger, sweating, odd behaviour, slow onset? — **No** → Paraesthesia? — **No** → Flushing on recovery? — **No**

Hunger, sweating, odd behaviour, slow onset? — **Yes** → Consider HYPOGLYCAEMIA → Is patient diabetic? — **No** → Glucose tolerance test followed by long fast may show insulinoma or reactive hypo-glycaemia

Is patient diabetic? — **Yes** → Adjust therapy

Paraesthesia? — **Yes** → Hypocalcaemia? — **Yes** → Treat cause

Hypocalcaemia? — **No** → Attacks associated with hyperventilation or recumbent position? → HYSTERICAL HYPERVENTILATION likely

Flushing on recovery? — **Yes** → Suggests STOKES ADAMS ATTACK → Suspect cardiac cause → Chest pain? — **Yes** → Exercise ECG may help → **No** → Go to 4

No (from associated features)

③ Could drug therapy be responsible? — **Yes** → Especially antihypertensives, diuretics, antianginal tranquillisers, chlorpromazine, antidepressants digoxin, levodopa

No

– see next page (3a)

6

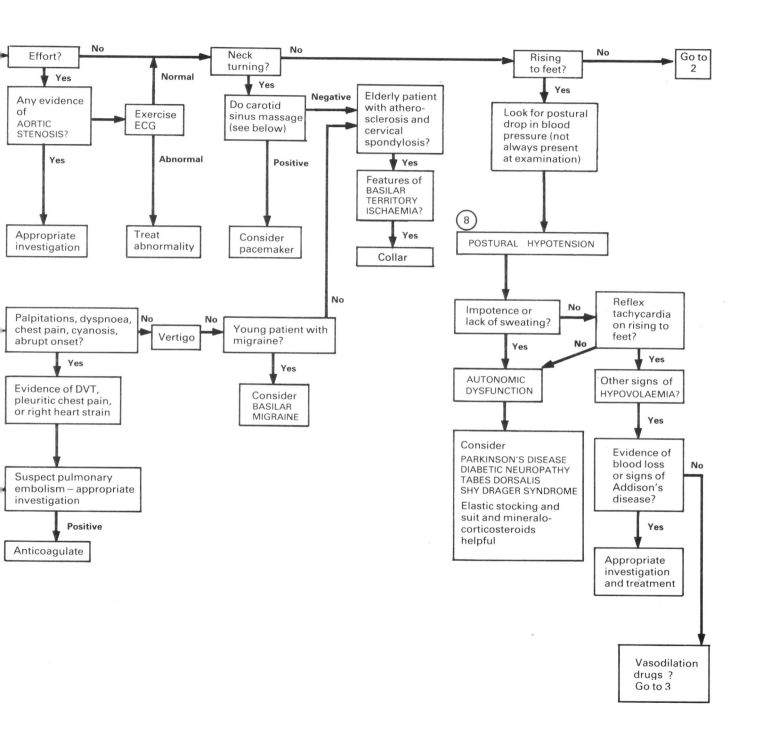

Effort? — No → Neck turning? — No → Rising to feet? — No → Go to 2

Effort? — Yes → Any evidence of AORTIC STENOSIS?

Any evidence of AORTIC STENOSIS? → Exercise ECG

Any evidence of AORTIC STENOSIS? — Yes → Appropriate investigation

Exercise ECG — Normal
Exercise ECG — Abnormal → Treat abnormality

Neck turning? — Yes → Do carotid sinus massage (see below)

Do carotid sinus massage (see below) — Negative → Elderly patient with athero-sclerosis and cervical spondylosis?

Do carotid sinus massage (see below) — Positive → Consider pacemaker

Elderly patient with athero-sclerosis and cervical spondylosis? — Yes → Features of BASILAR TERRITORY ISCHAEMIA?

Features of BASILAR TERRITORY ISCHAEMIA? — Yes → Collar

Rising to feet? — Yes → Look for postural drop in blood pressure (not always present at examination)

Look for postural drop in blood pressure → ⑧ POSTURAL HYPOTENSION

POSTURAL HYPOTENSION → Impotence or lack of sweating?

Impotence or lack of sweating? — No → Reflex tachycardia on rising to feet?

Impotence or lack of sweating? — Yes → AUTONOMIC DYSFUNCTION

Reflex tachycardia on rising to feet? — No → AUTONOMIC DYSFUNCTION
Reflex tachycardia on rising to feet? — Yes → Other signs of HYPOVOLAEMIA?

AUTONOMIC DYSFUNCTION → Consider
PARKINSON'S DISEASE
DIABETIC NEUROPATHY
TABES DORSALIS
SHY DRAGER SYNDROME

Elastic stocking and suit and mineralo-corticosteroids helpful

Other signs of HYPOVOLAEMIA? — Yes → Evidence of blood loss or signs of Addison's disease?

Evidence of blood loss or signs of Addison's disease? — Yes → Appropriate investigation and treatment

Evidence of blood loss or signs of Addison's disease? — No → Vasodilation drugs ? Go to 3

Palpitations, dyspnoea, chest pain, cyanosis, abrupt onset? — No → Vertigo

Vertigo — No → Young patient with migraine?

Young patient with migraine? — No (→ Elderly patient with athero-sclerosis...)

Young patient with migraine? — Yes → Consider BASILAR MIGRAINE

Palpitations, dyspnoea, chest pain, cyanosis, abrupt onset? — Yes → Evidence of DVT, pleuritic chest pain, or right heart strain

Evidence of DVT, pleuritic chest pain, or right heart strain → Suspect pulmonary embolism – appropriate investigation

Suspect pulmonary embolism – appropriate investigation — Positive → Anticoagulate

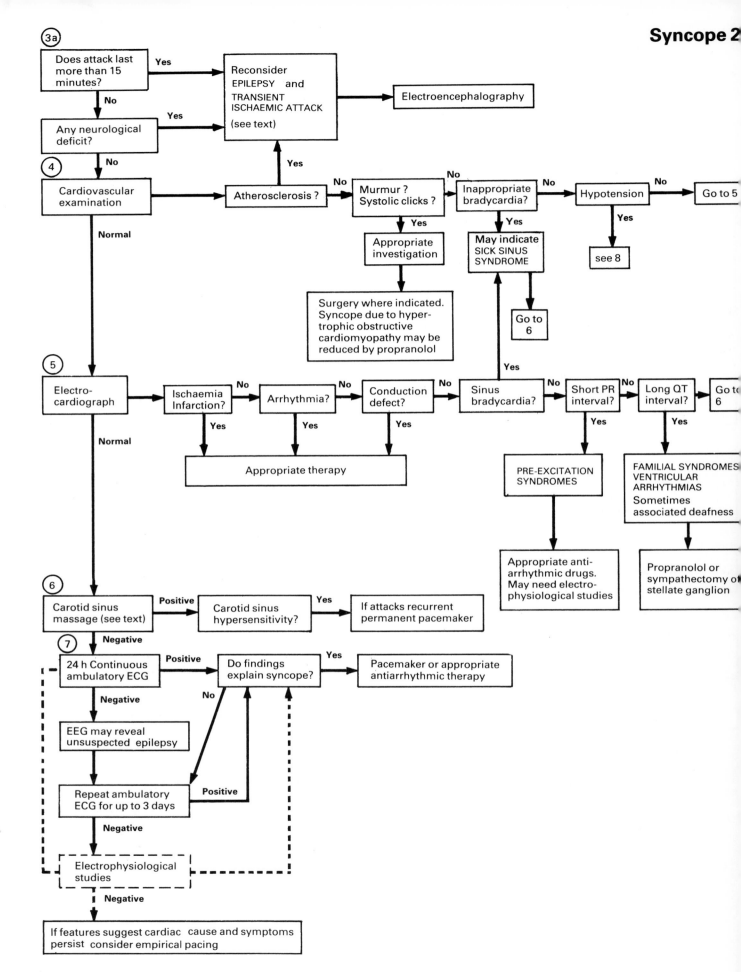

③a

Does attack last more than 15 minutes? — **Yes** → Reconsider EPILEPSY and TRANSIENT ISCHAEMIC ATTACK (see text) → Electroencephalography

No ↓

Any neurological deficit? — **Yes** → Reconsider EPILEPSY and TRANSIENT ISCHAEMIC ATTACK

No ↓

④ Cardiovascular examination → Atherosclerosis? — **Yes** ↑ (to Reconsider EPILEPSY)

Atherosclerosis? — **No** → Murmur ? Systolic clicks ? — **No** → Inappropriate bradycardia? — **No** → Hypotension — **No** → Go to 5

Murmur ? Systolic clicks ? — **Yes** ↓ Appropriate investigation ↓ Surgery where indicated. Syncope due to hypertrophic obstructive cardiomyopathy may be reduced by propranolol

Inappropriate bradycardia? — **Yes** ↓ May indicate SICK SINUS SYNDROME → Go to 6

Hypotension — **Yes** ↓ see 8

Cardiovascular examination — **Normal** ↓

⑤ Electro-cardiograph → Ischaemia Infarction? — **No** → Arrhythmia? — **No** → Conduction defect? — **No** → Sinus bradycardia? — **No** → Short PR interval? — **No** → Long QT interval? — Go to 6

Ischaemia Infarction? — **Yes** ↓ Appropriate therapy

Arrhythmia? — **Yes** ↓ Appropriate therapy

Conduction defect? — **Yes** ↓ Appropriate therapy

Sinus bradycardia? — **Yes** ↑ May indicate SICK SINUS SYNDROME

Short PR interval? — **Yes** ↓ PRE-EXCITATION SYNDROMES ↓ Appropriate anti-arrhythmic drugs. May need electro-physiological studies

Long QT interval? — **Yes** ↓ FAMILIAL SYNDROMES VENTRICULAR ARRHYTHMIAS Sometimes associated deafness ↓ Propranolol or sympathectomy of stellate ganglion

Electro-cardiograph — **Normal** ↓

⑥ Carotid sinus massage (see text) — **Positive** → Carotid sinus hypersensitivity? — **Yes** → If attacks recurrent permanent pacemaker

Carotid sinus massage (see text) — **Negative** ↓

⑦ 24 h Continuous ambulatory ECG — **Positive** → Do findings explain syncope? — **Yes** → Pacemaker or appropriate antiarrhythmic therapy

Do findings explain syncope? — **No** ↓

24 h Continuous ambulatory ECG — **Negative** ↓

EEG may reveal unsuspected epilepsy ↓

Repeat ambulatory ECG for up to 3 days — **Positive** → Do findings explain syncope?

Repeat ambulatory ECG for up to 3 days — **Negative** ↓

Electrophysiological studies — **Negative** ↓

If features suggest cardiac cause and symptoms persist consider empirical pacing

8

HEADACHE

M J JAMIESON

Headache, although a near universal experience, is a relatively uncommon reason for consultation in general practice. The consultation rate for migraine, for example, is said to be 12 per 1000 consultations, and it is estimated that the average general practitioner will see 28 patients on account of headache yearly.[1]

Most headache is of the migrainous or tension type. Fry estimates that less than 1% of headaches presenting to a general practitioner reflect "major intracranial disease."[2] Despite its predominantly benign nature, headache may, however, be the presenting feature of potentially serious conditions such as cerebral tumour, meningitis, giant cell arteritis, and glaucoma. Cervical spondylosis, chronic sinusitis, refractory errors, and hypertension probably cause headache less often than is commonly supposed.

Classification

A useful classification is that of the National Institute of Neurological Disease and Blindness 1962.[3] This is summarised below.

(1) Vascular headache of migraine type:
 A Classic migraine,
 B Common migraine,
 C Cluster headache,
 D Hemiplegic and ophthalmoplegic migraine,
 E "Lower half" headache.

(2) Muscle contraction headache.

(3) Combined headache: vascular and muscle contraction.

(4) Headache of nasal vasomotor reaction.

(5) Headache of delusional, conversional, or hypochondriacal states.

(6) Non-migrainous vascular headaches:
 A Systemic infections,
 B Miscellaneous disorders.

(7) Traction headache:
 A Primary or metastatic tumours of meninges, vessels, or brain,
 B Haematomas,
 C Abscesses,
 D Postlumbar puncture headache,
 E Pseudotumour cerebri.

(8) Headache due to overt cranial inflammation:
 A Intracranial,
 B Extracranial (arteritis, cellulitis).

(9) Headache due to disease of ocular structures.

(10) Headache due to disease of aural structures.

(11) Headache due to disease of nasal and sinusal structures.

(12) Headache due to disease of dental structures.

(13) Headache due to disease of other cranial and neck structures.

(14) Cranial neuritides (trauma, new growth, inflammation).

(15) Cranial neuralgias.

Diagnosis

History—Try to discover why the patient is presenting now. In many cases, particularly of acute onset headache, the reason will be clear. In a considerable proportion of cases of longstanding headache the consultation will have been precipitated by other factors. In particular, look for any underlying anxiety or depression. Attempt to elicit obvious pointers to specific causes (detailed in the classification and algorithm). From the history it is often not possible to differentiate serious from more benign causes. Features such as intensity, response to head movement and to vasoactive drugs, and the presence of a tender cervical spine with diminished movement do not have discriminating value. There are, however, certain uncommon alerting features, which again do not clearly discriminate but which should give rise to suspicion of in particular an expanding intracranial lesion. These are: (a) sleep disturbance, (b) paroxysmal headache, (c) cough headache.[4]

Examination—One cannot be dogmatic about the approach to examination in general practice. Nevertheless, it is reasonable to measure the blood pressure in all cases. In older patients examination of the superficial temporal arteries and of the intraocular tension would be appropriate. Examination will, on the whole, be guided by the history.

Investigations—There is no indication for routine investigation, other than the erythrocyte sedimentation rate in the older patient.

[1] Royal College of General Practitioners/Office of Population Censuses and Surveys 1974. *Morbidity statistics from general practice: second national study 1970-71.* London: HMSO, 1974. Studies on Medical and Population Subjects No 26.
[2] Fry J. *Common diseases, their nature, incidence and care.* 2nd ed. Lancaster: MTP Press Ltd, 1979.
[3] Vinken PJ, Bruyn GW. *Handbook of clinical neurology 5: headaches and cranial neuralgias.* Amsterdam: North Holland Publishing Company, 1968.
[4] Raskin NH, Appenzeller O. *Headache.* Philadelphia, WB Saunders, 1980. (Major problems in internal medicine; vol 19.)

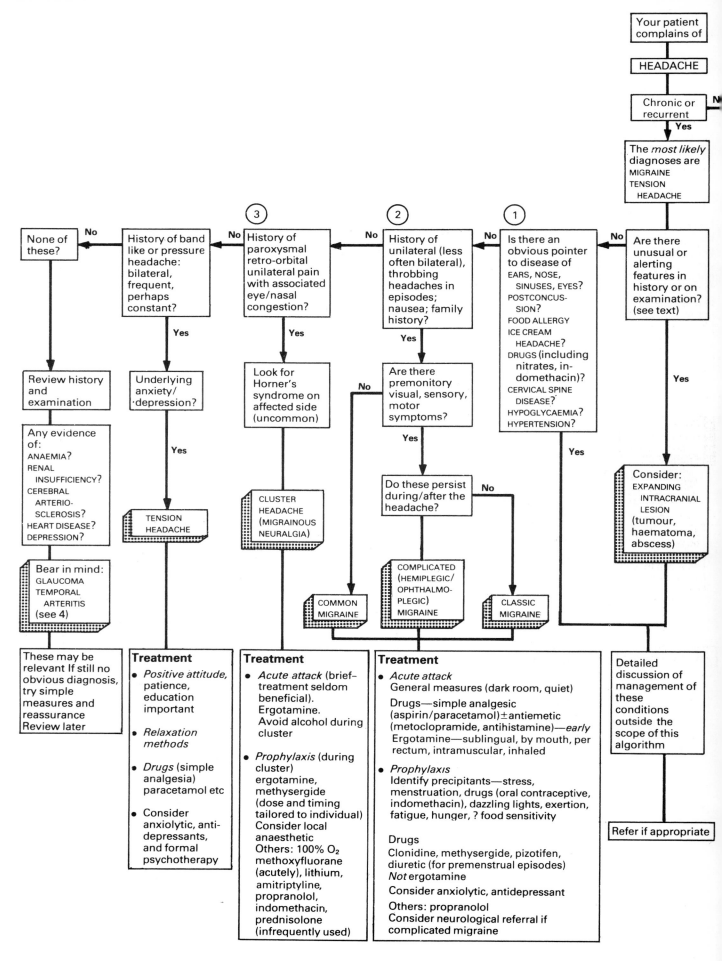

Your patient complains of

HEADACHE

Chronic or recurrent — **N**

Yes

The *most likely* diagnoses are
MIGRAINE
TENSION
    HEADACHE

① ② ③

No — Is there an obvious pointer to disease of
EARS, NOSE, SINUSES, EYES?
POSTCONCUSSION?
FOOD ALLERGY
ICE CREAM HEADACHE?
DRUGS (including nitrates, indomethacin)?
CERVICAL SPINE DISEASE?
HYPOGLYCAEMIA?
HYPERTENSION?

No — Are there unusual or alerting features in history or on examination? (see text)

Yes →

Consider:
EXPANDING INTRACRANIAL LESION (tumour, haematoma, abscess)

Detailed discussion of management of these conditions outside the scope of this algorithm

Refer if appropriate

② No — History of unilateral (less often bilateral), throbbing headaches in episodes; nausea; family history?

Yes

Are there premonitory visual, sensory, motor symptoms?

No →

Yes

Do these persist during/after the headache?

No →

COMPLICATED (HEMIPLEGIC/ OPHTHALMO-PLEGIC) MIGRAINE

COMMON MIGRAINE

CLASSIC MIGRAINE

Treatment
- *Acute attack*
  General measures (dark room, quiet)
  Drugs—simple analgesic (aspirin/paracetamol)±antiemetic (metoclopramide, antihistamine)—*early*
  Ergotamine—sublingual, by mouth, per rectum, intramuscular, inhaled
- *Prophylaxis*
  Identify precipitants—stress, menstruation, drugs (oral contraceptive, indomethacin), dazzling lights, exertion, fatigue, hunger, ? food sensitivity
  Drugs
  Clonidine, methysergide, pizotifen, diuretic (for premenstrual episodes)
  Not ergotamine
  Consider anxiolytic, antidepressant
  Others: propranolol
  Consider neurological referral if complicated migraine

② No — History of paroxysmal retro-orbital unilateral pain with associated eye/nasal congestion?

Yes

Look for Horner's syndrome on affected side (uncommon)

CLUSTER HEADACHE (MIGRAINOUS NEURALGIA)

Treatment
- *Acute attack* (brief-treatment seldom beneficial).
  Ergotamine.
  Avoid alcohol during cluster
- *Prophylaxis* (during cluster)
  ergotamine, methysergide (dose and timing tailored to individual)
  Consider local anaesthetic
  Others: 100% O₂ methoxyfluorane (acutely), lithium, amitriptyline, propranolol, indomethacin, prednisolone (infrequently used)

③ No — History of band like or pressure headache: bilateral, frequent, perhaps constant?

Yes

Underlying anxiety/depression?

Yes

TENSION HEADACHE

Treatment
- *Positive attitude,* patience, education important
- *Relaxation methods*
- *Drugs* (simple analgesia) paracetamol etc
- Consider anxiolytic, antidepressants, and formal psychotherapy

No — None of these?

Review history and examination

Any evidence of:
ANAEMIA?
RENAL INSUFFICIENCY?
CEREBRAL ARTERIO-SCLEROSIS?
HEART DISEASE?
DEPRESSION?

Bear in mind:
GLAUCOMA
TEMPORAL ARTERITIS
    (see 4)

These may be relevant If still no obvious diagnosis, try simple measures and reassurance Review later

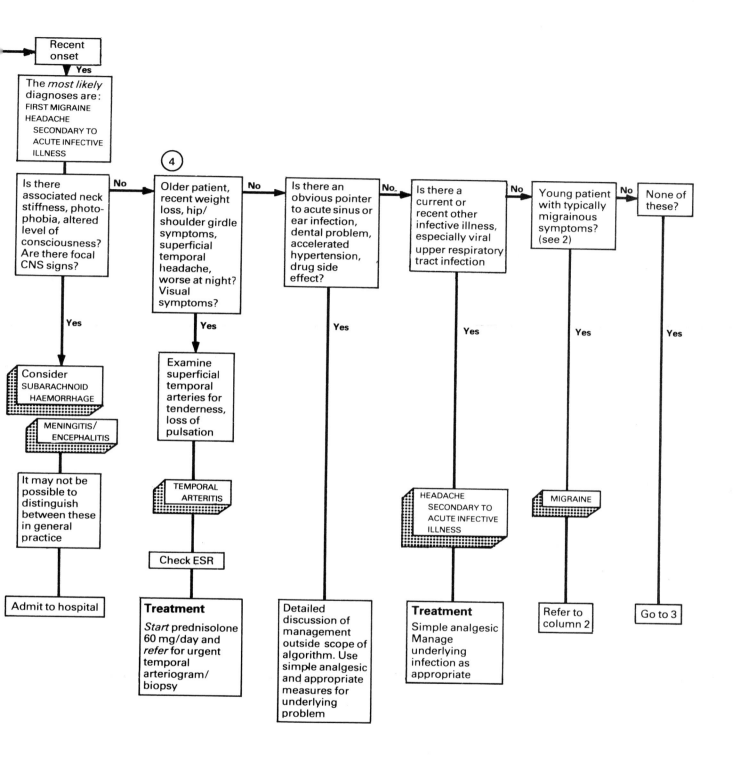

Recent onset

Yes →

The *most likely* diagnoses are:
FIRST MIGRAINE
HEADACHE
SECONDARY TO
ACUTE INFECTIVE
ILLNESS

④

Is there associated neck stiffness, photophobia, altered level of consciousness? Are there focal CNS signs? — **No** →

Older patient, recent weight loss, hip/shoulder girdle symptoms, superficial temporal headache, worse at night? Visual symptoms? — **No** →

Is there an obvious pointer to acute sinus or ear infection, dental problem, accelerated hypertension, drug side effect? — **No** →

Is there a current or recent other infective illness, especially viral upper respiratory tract infection — **No** →

Young patient with typically migrainous symptoms? (see 2) — **No** →

None of these?

Yes ↓ (under first box)

Consider
SUBARACHNOID
HAEMORRHAGE

MENINGITIS/
ENCEPHALITIS

It may not be possible to distinguish between these in general practice

Admit to hospital

Yes ↓ (under second box)

Examine superficial temporal arteries for tenderness, loss of pulsation

TEMPORAL
ARTERITIS

Check ESR

Treatment

Start prednisolone 60 mg/day and *refer* for urgent temporal arteriogram/biopsy

Yes ↓ (under third box)

Detailed discussion of management outside scope of algorithm. Use simple analgesic and appropriate measures for underlying problem

Yes ↓ (under fourth box)

HEADACHE
SECONDARY TO
ACUTE INFECTIVE
ILLNESS

Treatment

Simple analgesic Manage underlying infection as appropriate

Yes ↓ (under fifth box)

MIGRAINE

Refer to column 2

Yes ↓ (under sixth box)

Go to 3

SENSORY DISTURBANCES

DAVID I SHEPHERD

In clinical practice patients often complain of sensory disturbance, but arriving at a satisfactory diagnosis may be difficult. The complaint is subjective and our ability to test objectively is limited. The tools of the trade comprise a pin, preferably disposable, and certainly not a hypodermic needle, which penetrates the skin; cottonwool; a tuning fork 128 Hz (not 256 or 512 Hz, which are preferable for testing hearing), which can also serve to test cold sensation; and a two point discriminator (two orange sticks can be equally effective). Despite judicious use of these implements, however, in many patients complaining of numbness no abnormality can be found. This simply reflects our inability to test the function of many of the fibres carrying sensation.

Points to note

(1) Continuous sensory disturbance affecting a given area is more important than transient symptoms except in stereotyped conditions, such as the nocturnal paraesthesiae of the carpal tunnel syndrome.

(2) A band like sensation is usually important and reflects dorsal column disturbance.

(3) Electric-like tingling sensations also originate in the dorsal columns, perhaps best typified by Lhermitte's sign, which can occur in subacute combined degeneration, cervical spondylosis, and tumour, as well as in multiple sclerosis.

(4) A deep aching pain can reflect spinothalamic involvement.

(5) Physiological areas of increased sensitivity are present at the groin, costal margin, and where the supraclavicular nerves border on the T2 dermatome over the upper chest. If this is not recognised one may assume wrongly that sensory abnormalities are present below these levels.

(6) Hyperaesthesia can reflect sensory disturbance just as much as hypoaesthesia.

(7) Trigeminal sensory upset should stop above the angle of the jaw.

(8) T2 dermatone does run down the inner aspect of the upper arm.

(9) In joint position sense testing the patient has a 50% chance of being correct. A significant deficit will be present, however, if it takes more than 5 mm of movement before the patient appreciates it.

(10) Pseudoathetoid movements of the outstretched fingers often reflect disturbance of the posterior column, although the patient may have little in the way of sensory complaint. This most often occurs in cervical spondylotic myelopathy and multiple sclerosis.

(11) Testing two point discrimination, vibration, and joint position sense is less subjective than testing for pinprick, temperature, and touch.

(12) If the patient does not complain of sensory disturbance it is unlikely that a major deficit is present, although there are exceptions.

(13) A dorsal column lesion may be associated with the loss of both vibration sense and joint position sense, whereas a lesion of the cortex is usually associated only with impairment of joint position sense.

Distinguishing organic and non-organic sensory disturbance

(1) With a definite sensory level there is usually an area of altered sensation between the normal and abnormal. In a non-organic condition the transition is sudden.

(2) Hysterical sensory loss does not follow the line of dermatomal distribution, which dips anteriorly on the trunk.

(3) In hysterical disturbance in a limb there may be total loss of vibration sense but normal joint position sense, or pinprick loss but preserved temperature sensation. In addition, pseudoathetoid movements are usually absent despite gross posterior column disturbance.

(4) In organic spinothalamic loss a cut off circumferentially at the groin or armpit is exceptional.

When considering a patient with sensory disturbance, it is important to think anatomically since this should provide the vital clues to the cause. See chart.

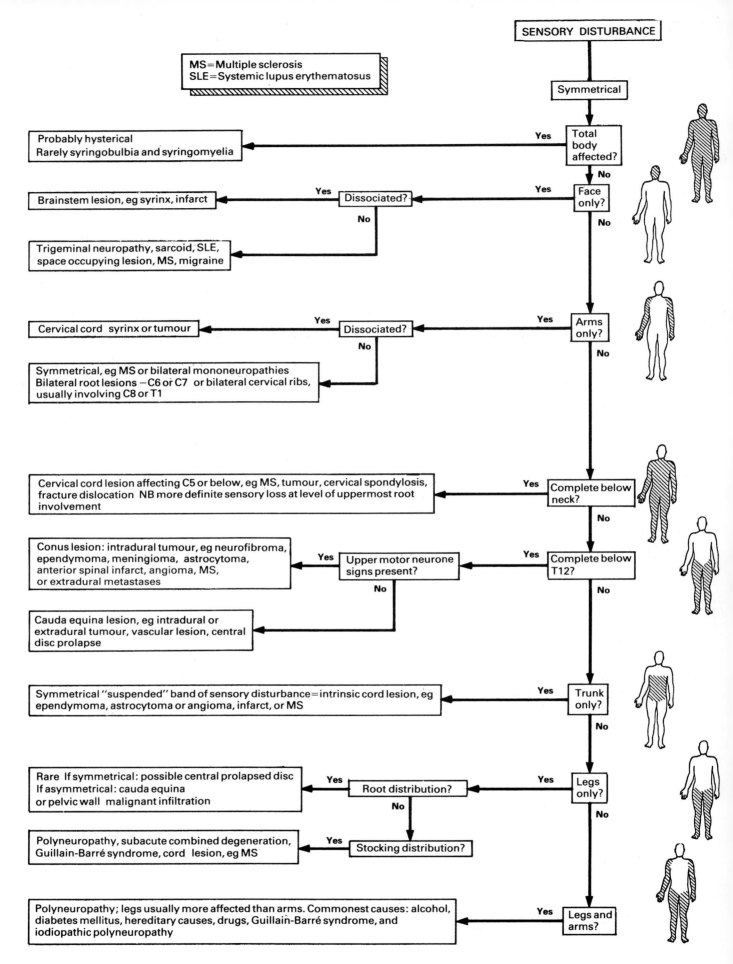

SENSORY DISTURBANCE

Symmetrical

MS=Multiple sclerosis
SLE=Systemic lupus erythematosus

Total body affected? — Yes → Probably hysterical. Rarely syringobulbia and syringomyelia

No ↓

Face only? — Yes → **Dissociated?** — Yes → Brainstem lesion, eg syrinx, infarct

No → Trigeminal neuropathy, sarcoid, SLE, space occupying lesion, MS, migraine

No ↓

Arms only? — Yes → **Dissociated?** — Yes → Cervical cord syrinx or tumour

No → Symmetrical, eg MS or bilateral mononeuropathies. Bilateral root lesions —C6 or C7 or bilateral cervical ribs, usually involving C8 or T1

No ↓

Complete below neck? — Yes → Cervical cord lesion affecting C5 or below, eg MS, tumour, cervical spondylosis, fracture dislocation NB more definite sensory loss at level of uppermost root involvement

No ↓

Complete below T12? — Yes → **Upper motor neurone signs present?** — Yes → Conus lesion: intradural tumour, eg neurofibroma, ependymoma, meningioma, astrocytoma, anterior spinal infarct, angioma, MS, or extradural metastases

No → Cauda equina lesion, eg intradural or extradural tumour, vascular lesion, central disc prolapse

No ↓

Trunk only? — Yes → Symmetrical "suspended" band of sensory disturbance=intrinsic cord lesion, eg ependymoma, astrocytoma or angioma, infarct, or MS

No ↓

Legs only? — Yes → **Root distribution?** — Yes → Rare If symmetrical: possible central prolapsed disc If asymmetrical: cauda equina or pelvic wall malignant infiltration

No → **Stocking distribution?** — Yes → Polyneuropathy, subacute combined degeneration, Guillain-Barré syndrome, cord lesion, eg MS

No ↓

Legs and arms? — Yes → Polyneuropathy; legs usually more affected than arms. Commonest causes: alcohol, diabetes mellitus, hereditary causes, drugs, Guillain-Barré syndrome, and iodiopathic polyneuropathy

14

Sensory disturbances

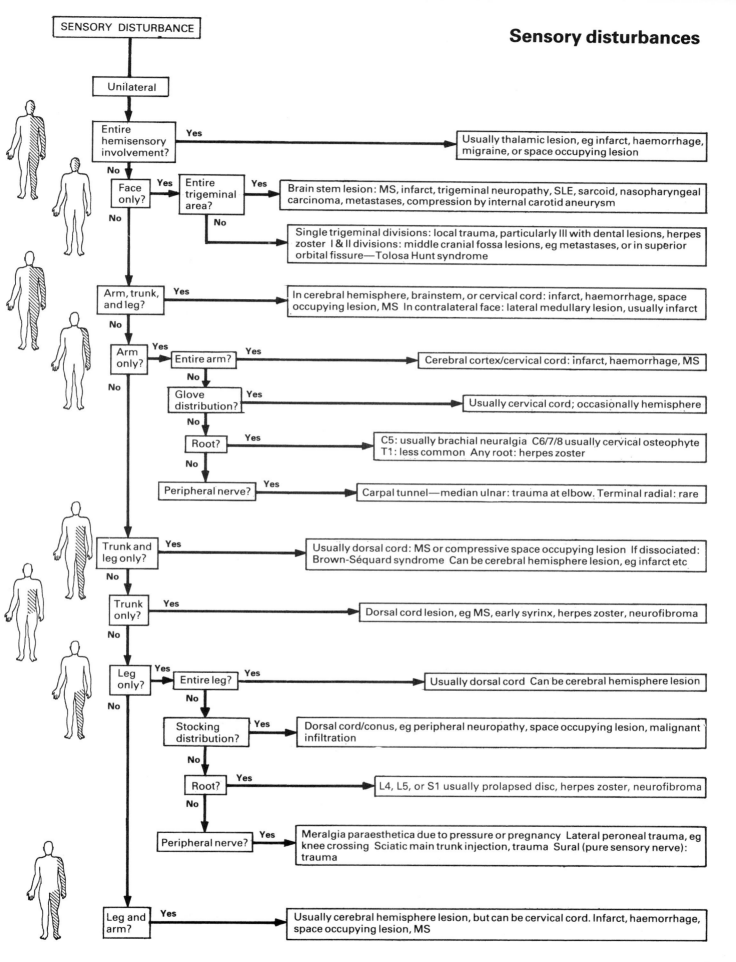

SENSORY DISTURBANCE

Unilateral

Entire hemisensory involvement? — Yes → Usually thalamic lesion, eg infarct, haemorrhage, migraine, or space occupying lesion

No

Face only? — Yes → **Entire trigeminal area?** — Yes → Brain stem lesion: MS, infarct, trigeminal neuropathy, SLE, sarcoid, nasopharyngeal carcinoma, metastases, compression by internal carotid aneurysm

No → Single trigeminal divisions: local trauma, particularly III with dental lesions, herpes zoster I & II divisions: middle cranial fossa lesions, eg metastases, or in superior orbital fissure—Tolosa Hunt syndrome

No

Arm, trunk, and leg? — Yes → In cerebral hemisphere, brainstem, or cervical cord: infarct, haemorrhage, space occupying lesion, MS In contralateral face: lateral medullary lesion, usually infarct

No

Arm only? — Yes → **Entire arm?** — Yes → Cerebral cortex/cervical cord: infarct, haemorrhage, MS

No

Glove distribution? — Yes → Usually cervical cord; occasionally hemisphere

No

Root? — Yes → C5: usually brachial neuralgia C6/7/8 usually cervical osteophyte T1: less common Any root: herpes zoster

No

Peripheral nerve? — Yes → Carpal tunnel—median ulnar: trauma at elbow. Terminal radial: rare

No

Trunk and leg only? — Yes → Usually dorsal cord: MS or compressive space occupying lesion If dissociated: Brown-Séquard syndrome Can be cerebral hemisphere lesion, eg infarct etc

No

Trunk only? — Yes → Dorsal cord lesion, eg MS, early syrinx, herpes zoster, neurofibroma

No

Leg only? — Yes → **Entire leg?** — Yes → Usually dorsal cord Can be cerebral hemisphere lesion

No

Stocking distribution? — Yes → Dorsal cord/conus, eg peripheral neuropathy, space occupying lesion, malignant infiltration

No

Root? — Yes → L4, L5, or S1 usually prolapsed disc, herpes zoster, neurofibroma

No

Peripheral nerve? — Yes → Meralgia paraesthetica due to pressure or pregnancy Lateral peroneal trauma, eg knee crossing Sciatic main trunk injection, trauma Sural (pure sensory nerve): trauma

No

Leg and arm? — Yes → Usually cerebral hemisphere lesion, but can be cervical cord. Infarct, haemorrhage, space occupying lesion, MS

DIZZINESS AND VERTIGO

HAMISH M A TOWLER

Dizziness and vertigo are common complaints. The terms cover various sensations, and the distinction between the two is not clear. Careful inquiry into the patient's history is of paramount importance as this may establish the diagnosis when examination yields normal results.

Vertigo indicates vestibular dysfunction and is usually defined as a sense of rotation of either the patient or his environment. This rigid definition, however, excludes patients with vestibular dysfunction who feel only a sensation of imbalance or disequilibrium in the head. Imbalance felt in the legs usually results from a cerebellar or proprioceptive deficit or from weakness of the legs.

Dizziness, a feeling of impending loss of consciousness, is usually vascular in origin. Postural hypotension, cardiac dysrrhythmia such as in Adams-Stokes disease, low cardiac output resulting from valvular disease, or ventricular dysfunction may all present in this manner. The remainder of patients with dizziness may describe their symptoms in vague terms, such as "light headedness," "a fear of falling," or "a swimming sensation"; a common aetiology here is emotional disturbance.

Vertigo of acute onset, and particularly when the labyrinth is affected, is characteristically rotatory and often associated with constitutional upset such as nausea, vomiting, or sweating. If the onset is gradual central compensation can occur and disequilibrium is the predominant complaint. The clinician should ask about symptoms of middle ear disease, deafness, tinnitus, headache, or focal neurological dysfunction and ascertain whether symptoms are provoked by specific movements—for example, of the head or neck—or changes of posture. The duration of symptoms and any particular pattern of recurrence should be established.

Many drugs may cause dizziness and, less commonly, vertigo. Drugs that are directly vestibulotoxic, such as aminoglycosides, tend to cause disequilibrium as damage is predominantly bilateral. Rotatory vertigo, however, may occasionally develop as a result of unilateral toxicity. The inappropriate use of labyrinthine sedatives may aggravate dizziness, particularly in elderly people.

Examination should be directed by history. Anaemia or polycythaemia may be apparent. The ears should be carefully examined, hearing tested, and tuning fork tests performed. The eyes should be examined closely for nystagmus or ocular paresis and the pupillary responses and corneal reflexes tested. Fundoscopy may show such abnormalities as papilloedema, papillitis, or optic atrophy.

Positional testing for nystagmus and vertigo should be performed as follows. The patient sits upright on a couch with his gaze fixed on the examiner's forehead; his head is then briskly and simultaneously rotated through 45° and lowered to 30° below horizontal beyond the end of the couch. Both directions of rotation are tested and the eyes scrutinised for nystagmus. There are two positive responses. Most commonly, severe vertigo and nystagmus towards the lower ear develop after a latent period, then fatigue within 30 seconds. On repeat testing adaptation occurs: both vertigo and nystagmus are diminished. This is benign paroxysmal vertigo, which is caused by a peripheral disorder of the bottom most labyrinth. In the other pattern of response nystagmus develops immediately on provocation, with no latent period, there is no fatigue or adaptation, and vertigo is usually mild or absent. Here the lesion is central, usually a posterior fossa tumour or, less commonly, vascular disease or multiple sclerosis. The other cranial nerves should also be tested. There may be evidence of long tract motor or sensory damage or peripheral neuropathy. Gait should be observed and the patient tested for rombergism. Truncal ataxia on heel toe walking may be the only clinical evidence of midline cerebellar disease causing disequilibrium.

Cardiovascular examination may show dysrrhythmia, valvular disease (particularly aortic stenosis), carotid or vertebral bruits, or cardiac failure. Erect and supine blood pressure must be measured. Disease of the middle or inner ear or focal neurological signs in a patient with vertigo merits prompt referral. Further investigations to establish the diagnosis may include audiometry, caloric testing, electronystagmography, and advanced radiology. Such cases are, however, rare.

The commonest cause of acute vertigo in young people is sudden vestibular failure (acute labyrinthitis), possibly due to recent viral infection. It may also be caused by head injury, migraine, or multiple sclerosis and, in older patients, vertebrobasilar disease. Transient ischaemic attacks or infarction in the vertebrobasilar territory rarely cause vertigo or tinnitus without other focal neurological symptoms such as diplopia, dysarthria, weakness, or sensory disturbance. In patients aged over 50 benign positional vertigo is more common than Menière's disease, though Menière's disease is often mistakenly diagnosed. The main features of Menière's disease are recurrent paroxysms of vertigo, tinnitus, and progressive hearing loss. Cervical spondylosis is common in old people and too often blamed for symptoms. It should be considered only when vertigo is clearly associated with movements of the neck (not the head) and appreciable radiological changes. Vasculitis may simulate vertebrobasilar arteriosclerosis, and, although they are rare, cranial arteritis, polyarteritis nodosum, systemic lupus erythematosus, and syphilis should not be forgotten.

Acoustic neuromas and other tumours of the cerebellopontine angle are rare and cause unilateral deafness and tinnitus initially, disequilibrium less often, and rotatory vertigo only when well advanced. Impairment of the corneal reflex is an important sign, but small tumours are identified only if there is a strong index of suspicion in patients with unilateral sensorineural deafness and prompt referral for investigation.

Psychiatric and emotional problems are a common cause of dizziness. Hyperventilation can be confirmed if the patient's symptoms are provoked by voluntary overbreathing for three minutes. Chronic continuous dizziness may be a sign of depressive illness. Emotional factors may influence symptoms of organic origin—for example, stress may provoke bouts of Menière's disease as it does asthma and migraine.

Further reading

Drachman AA, Hart CW. An approach to the dizzy patient. *Neurology* 1972;**22**:323-34.
Finestone AJ, ed. *Evaluation and clinical management of dizziness and vertigo*. Bristol: John Wright, 1982.
Hibbert GA. Hyperventilation as a cause of panic attacks. *Br Med J* 1984;**288**:263-4.
Ludman H. *ABC of ENT*. London: BMA, 1981.
Luxon LM. Dizziness in the elderly. In: Hinchcliffe R, ed. *Hearing and balance in the elderly*. Edinburgh: Churchill Livingstone, 1983:402-52.
Yatsu FM, Smith JD. Neurologic aspects of vertigo. In: Ballantyne J, Groves J, eds. *Scott Brown's diseases of the ear, nose and throat*. Volume 2. 4th ed. Sevenoaks: Butterworths, 1979: 837-64.

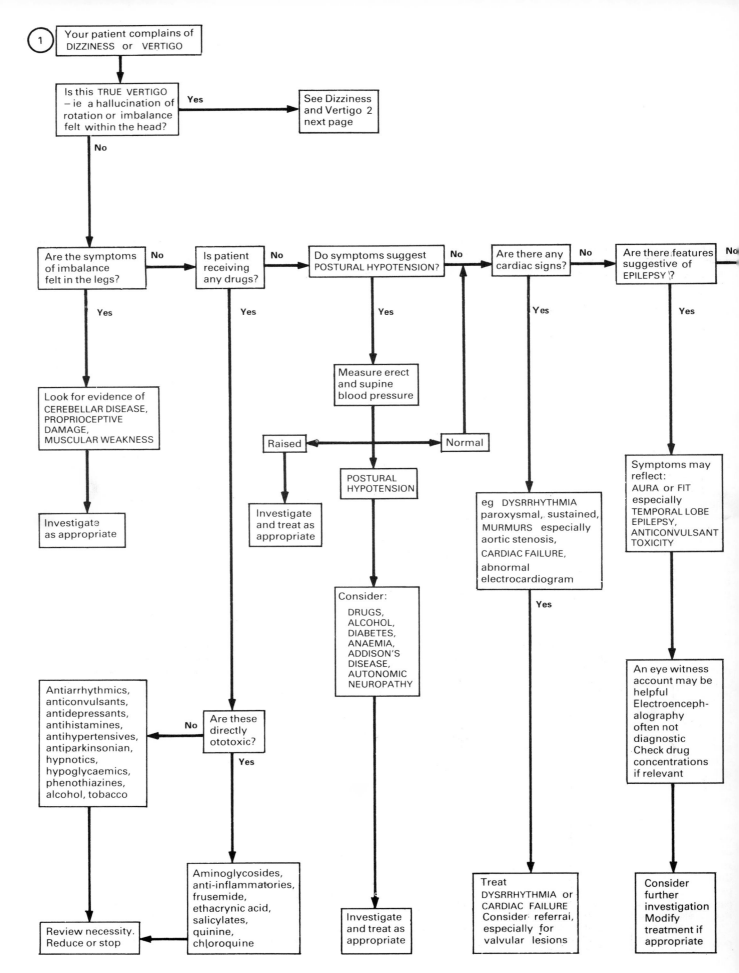

1 Your patient complains of DIZZINESS or VERTIGO

Is this TRUE VERTIGO – ie a hallucination of rotation or imbalance felt within the head? → **Yes** → See Dizziness and Vertigo 2 next page

No

Are the symptoms of imbalance felt in the legs? → **No** → Is patient receiving any drugs? → **No** → Do symptoms suggest POSTURAL HYPOTENSION? → **No** → Are there any cardiac signs? → **No** → Are there features suggestive of EPILEPSY? → **No**

Yes (imbalance in legs) ↓

Look for evidence of CEREBELLAR DISEASE, PROPRIOCEPTIVE DAMAGE, MUSCULAR WEAKNESS

Investigate as appropriate

Yes (drugs) ↓

Are these directly ototoxic?

No →

Antiarrhythmics, anticonvulsants, antidepressants, antihistamines, antihypertensives, antiparkinsonian, hypnotics, hypoglycaemics, phenothiazines, alcohol, tobacco

Yes ↓

Aminoglycosides, anti-inflammatories, frusemide, ethacrynic acid, salicylates, quinine, chloroquine

Review necessity. Reduce or stop

Yes (postural hypotension) ↓

Measure erect and supine blood pressure

Raised ← → Normal

POSTURAL HYPOTENSION

Investigate and treat as appropriate (Raised)

Consider:
DRUGS, ALCOHOL, DIABETES, ANAEMIA, ADDISON'S DISEASE, AUTONOMIC NEUROPATHY

Investigate and treat as appropriate

Yes (cardiac signs) ↓

eg DYSRRHYTHMIA paroxysmal, sustained, MURMURS especially aortic stenosis, CARDIAC FAILURE, abnormal electrocardiogram

Yes ↓

Treat DYSRRHYTHMIA or CARDIAC FAILURE Consider referral, especially for valvular lesions

Yes (epilepsy) ↓

Symptoms may reflect: AURA or FIT especially TEMPORAL LOBE EPILEPSY, ANTICONVULSANT TOXICITY

An eye witness account may be helpful Electroencephalography often not diagnostic Check drug concentrations if relevant

Consider further investigation Modify treatment if appropriate

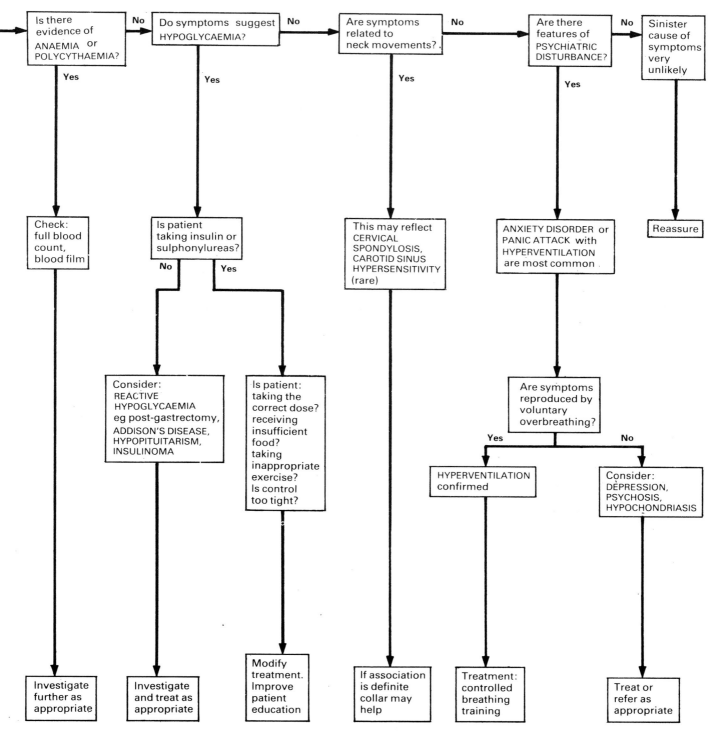

Is there evidence of ANAEMIA or POLYCYTHAEMIA? — No → **Do symptoms suggest HYPOGLYCAEMIA?** — No → **Are symptoms related to neck movements?** — No → **Are there features of PSYCHIATRIC DISTURBANCE?** — No → **Sinister cause of symptoms very unlikely**

Yes ↓ (Is there evidence...)
Check: full blood count, blood film
↓
Investigate further as appropriate

Yes ↓ (Do symptoms suggest HYPOGLYCAEMIA?)
Is patient taking insulin or sulphonylureas?
No ↓ — Yes ↓

No →
Consider: REACTIVE HYPOGLYCAEMIA eg post-gastrectomy, ADDISON'S DISEASE, HYPOPITUITARISM, INSULINOMA
↓
Investigate and treat as appropriate

Yes →
Is patient: taking the correct dose? receiving insufficient food? taking inappropriate exercise? Is control too tight?
↓
Modify treatment. Improve patient education

Yes ↓ (Are symptoms related to neck movements?)
This may reflect CERVICAL SPONDYLOSIS, CAROTID SINUS HYPERSENSITIVITY (rare)
↓
If association is definite collar may help

Yes ↓ (Are there features of PSYCHIATRIC DISTURBANCE?)
ANXIETY DISORDER or PANIC ATTACK with HYPERVENTILATION are most common
↓
Are symptoms reproduced by voluntary overbreathing?
Yes ↓ — No ↓

Yes →
HYPERVENTILATION confirmed
↓
Treatment: controlled breathing training

No →
Consider: DEPRESSION, PSYCHOSIS, HYPOCHONDRIASIS
↓
Treat or refer as appropriate

↓ (Sinister cause...)
Reassure

19

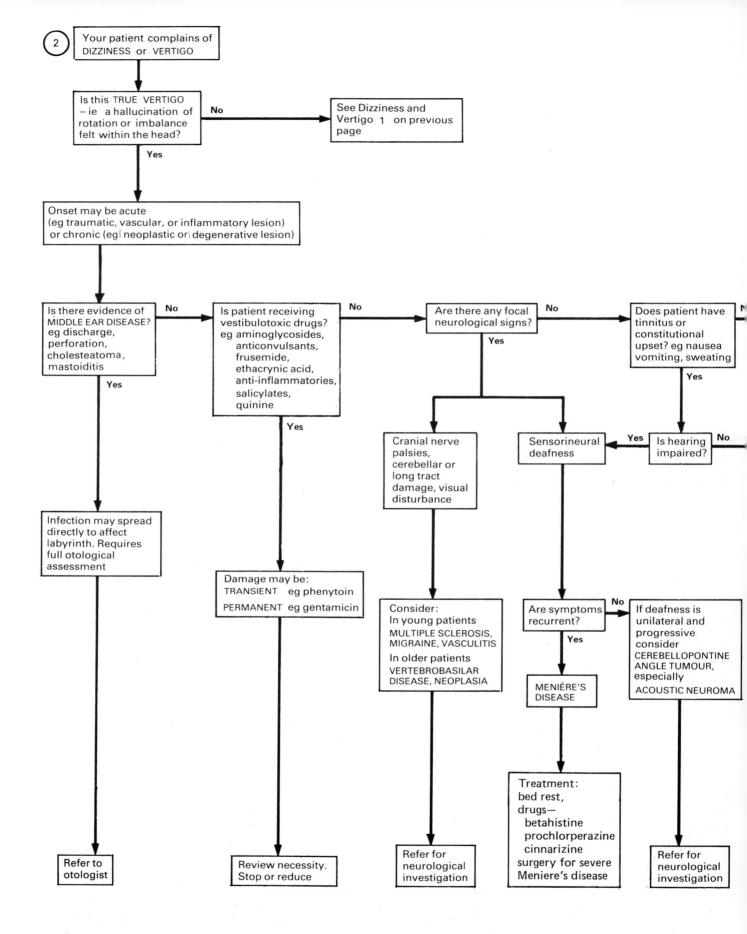

2 Your patient complains of DIZZINESS or VERTIGO

Is this TRUE VERTIGO – ie a hallucination of rotation or imbalance felt within the head? — **No** → See Dizziness and Vertigo 1 on previous page

Yes

Onset may be acute (eg traumatic, vascular, or inflammatory lesion) or chronic (eg neoplastic or degenerative lesion)

Is there evidence of MIDDLE EAR DISEASE? eg discharge, perforation, cholesteatoma, mastoiditis — **No** → Is patient receiving vestibulotoxic drugs? eg aminoglycosides, anticonvulsants, frusemide, ethacrynic acid, anti-inflammatories, salicylates, quinine — **No** → Are there any focal neurological signs? — **No** → Does patient have tinnitus or constitutional upset? eg nausea vomiting, sweating

Yes (Middle ear)

Yes (drugs)

Yes (neurological)

Yes (tinnitus)

Infection may spread directly to affect labyrinth. Requires full otological assessment

Damage may be:
TRANSIENT eg phenytoin
PERMANENT eg gentamicin

Cranial nerve palsies, cerebellar or long tract damage, visual disturbance

Sensorineural deafness ← **Yes** — Is hearing impaired? — **No**

Consider:
In young patients
MULTIPLE SCLEROSIS, MIGRAINE, VASCULITIS
In older patients
VERTEBROBASILAR DISEASE, NEOPLASIA

Are symptoms recurrent? — **No** → If deafness is unilateral and progressive consider CEREBELLOPONTINE ANGLE TUMOUR, especially ACOUSTIC NEUROMA

Yes

MENIÈRE'S DISEASE

Treatment:
bed rest,
drugs—
betahistine
prochlorperazine
cinnarizine
surgery for severe
Meniere's disease

Refer to otologist

Review necessity. Stop or reduce

Refer for neurological investigation

Refer for neurological investigation

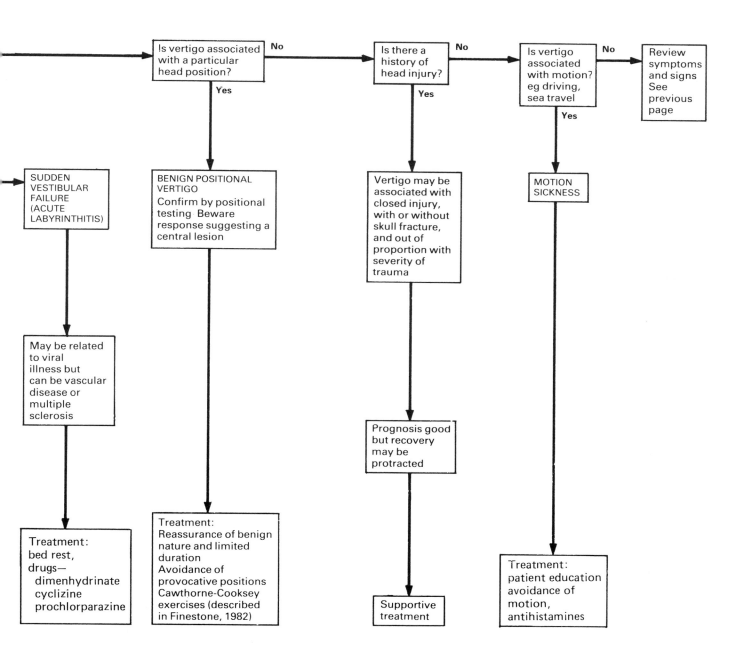

Is vertigo associated with a particular head position?

No → Is there a history of head injury?

No → Is vertigo associated with motion? eg driving, sea travel

No → Review symptoms and signs See previous page

Yes (head position) ↓

Yes (head injury) ↓

Yes (motion) ↓

SUDDEN VESTIBULAR FAILURE (ACUTE LABYRINTHITIS)

BENIGN POSITIONAL VERTIGO
Confirm by positional testing Beware response suggesting a central lesion

Vertigo may be associated with closed injury, with or without skull fracture, and out of proportion with severity of trauma

MOTION SICKNESS

May be related to viral illness but can be vascular disease or multiple sclerosis

Prognosis good but recovery may be protracted

Treatment:
bed rest,
drugs—
  dimenhydrinate
  cyclizine
  prochlorparazine

Treatment:
Reassurance of benign nature and limited duration
Avoidance of provocative positions
Cawthorne-Cooksey exercises (described in Finestone, 1982)

Supportive treatment

Treatment:
patient education avoidance of motion, antihistamines

21

MEMORY LOSS

ROBERT A WOOD

Memory loss covers a wide range of medicine, neurology, and psychiatry. This account touches on various conditions in which memory loss is only part of the picture, but I have emphasised pure amnesic states or others in which amnesic symptoms can occur early in the course of the illness. The importance lies in the early recognition of the treatable and in preventing deterioration where the cause is not inexorably progressive. The main subdivision is between amnesia of sudden onset, in which the outcome is usually favourable, and slow onset amnesia—often with global dementia—where it is not.

Memory

Defects of memory are either in the registration of new experience (antegrade) or the recall of past experience (retrograde). In gross dementia the patient may lose the ability to repeat a series of numbers he has just heard. This immediate type of defect is also seen in dysphasia, or whenever attention or concentration is distracted—as in depression or acute confusional states. Short term memory deficit is tested by inviting the recall of a few numbers and two or three names after five minutes of other conversation. The limbic system, including the mamillary bodies and hippocampus, must be intact for new experience to be registered and recent events recollected. In Korsakow's amnesia, where the main damage is in the mamillary bodies, antegrade amnesia—learning ability—is permanently damaged and several years of experience are lost. After head injury an antegrade defect is noted but this is temporary. The retrograde amnesia shrinks until minutes or seconds before the accident. Deep memory, including childhood events, can be retained and recalled when limbic structures no longer function. The long term memory is tested by asking for details of the patient and his family and about important people or events. Moments of great personal pleasure or poignancy can be recalled most clearly.

Alcohol related amnesia

When the blood alcohol concentration is very high the memory may be blacked out. This is impossible in inexperienced drinkers, who will pass out before they become amnesic. Many episodes of acute alcoholic amnesia lead on to delirium tremens, the withdrawal syndrome of alcohol tolerance, which is characterised by motor excitation, tremor, and hallucination; it clears within two to three days. Treatment is with chlormethiazole or haloperidol to reduce the excitation and with parenteral vitamin B complex to prevent the development of Wernicke's encephalopathy. Alcohol and its subsequent withdrawal are important causes of seizure in epileptics. Alcohol and head injury are often associated, and intracerebral clot is hard to diagnose in intoxicated or delirious alcoholics.

When prolonged drinking gives way to confusion, the presence of ataxia and diplopia or disorders of gaze indicate the development of Wernicke's encephalopathy. This confusional state is caused by thiamine deficiency. It should be suspected if the confusion of withdrawal does not clear in the usual time. If treatment with parenteral vitamin B complex is omitted or delayed a dense and permanent

Korsakow's amnesia will become apparent when the confusion clears. No treatment is worth while at this stage, and fewer than a tenth of patients show any improvement in the long term. Institutional care is the usual end result.

Chronic alcoholic dementia is more common than Korsakow's amnesia. The early features are occasionally amnesic, but generally judgment and social projection are impaired first. It is a long term toxic effect, usually in the older age groups, and the older the patient the poorer the prospect for improvement. Computed tomography usually shows cortical atrophy and ventricular enlargement; these may improve with abstinence, but the dementia itself seldom disappears entirely, and improvement is maximal after a month or two. Abstinence is the only beneficial treatment. This is the fourth most common progressive dementia.

Malingering and hysteria

Hysterical amnesia is rare. The patient may seem to remember nothing or forget only specific personal events. Feigned amnesia is common, often to avoid arrest or conviction: the subject who "disappears" after a car crash and turns up uninjured hours later has been hiding with the purpose of metabolising alcohol. It should be distinguished from the brief, complex, automatic activity seen in some temporal lobe seizures. The conscious non-dysphasic patient who cannot give his name does not have an organic diagnosis. Hysteria resolves in time.

Epilepsy

After a major seizure consciousness is recovered quickly but antegrade amnesia lasts for up to an hour. The patient may also appear muddled. Epilepsy is high on the list of possibilities in a patient who has been briefly amnesic and who has unaccountable injuries. In the known epileptic alcohol and failure to comply with prescribed drugs are common provocative factors. Epilepsy may occur in most of the organic syndromes in which amnesia occurs and both it and the medication used to control it may give a false impression of the severity of amnesia.

Post-traumatic brain syndrome

After head injury a classic amnesic syndrome is seen with severity and duration relating to the severity of injury. Most patients recover fully, though it may be days or weeks before the short term memory is restored. The retrograde amnesia, initially quite long in many patients, shrinks progressively until it is just seconds or minutes before the injury; this contrasts with the lengthy retrograde amnesia in Korsakow's syndrome.

The importance of the amnesia is that it confirms brain injury. Skull radiographs are useful, although a fractured skull is no predictor of the severity of the neurological injury. Computed tomography has revolutionised the management of head injury. Unconscious patients need specialised supervision in units where

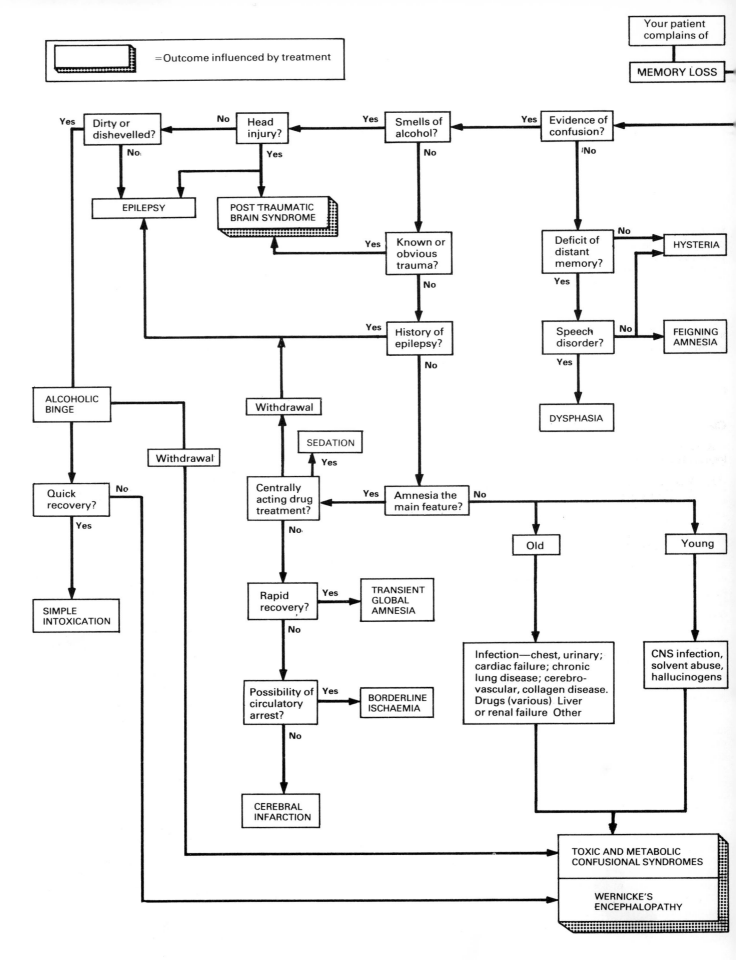

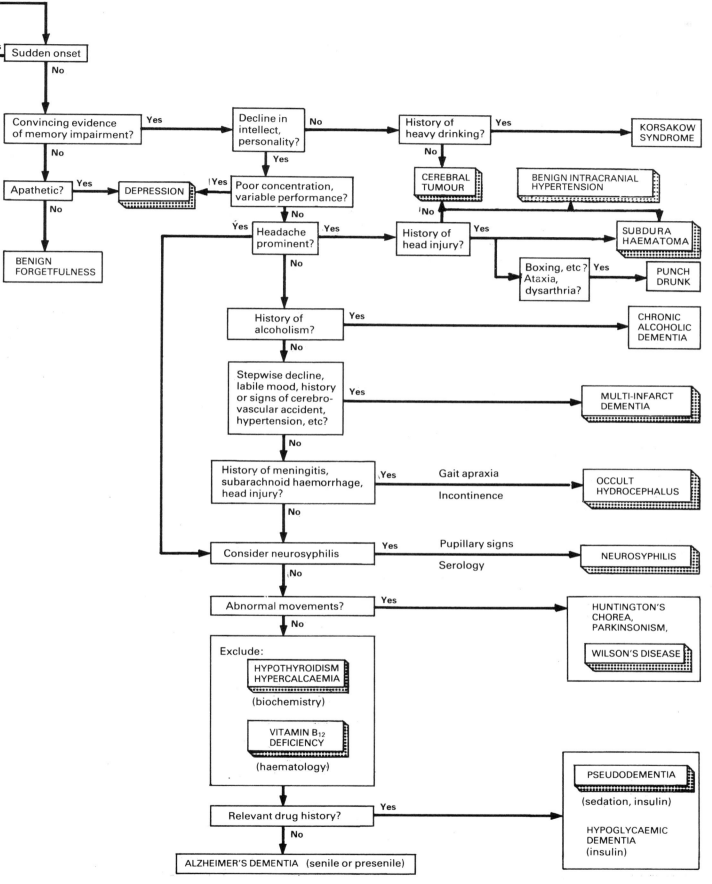

Memory Loss

the brain can be decompressed and the clot evacuated. Dexamethasone may reduce the duration of the organic brain syndrome after head injury or neurosurgery. Opiates and sedatives are unsuitable because of possible effects on eye signs and consciousness.

Cerebrovascular syndromes

Pure amnesia may be due to cerebrovascular disease. Transient global amnesia is common; memory for recent events is lost, usually for a few hours during which the patient can carry out various routine activities but has to be reminded that he has done so. Embolism or transient ischaemia in the basilar distribution is the likely cause; this may lead to temporary left hippocampal dysfunction. Full recovery occurs without treatment.

Rarely a cerebral infarct in the left hippocampus may produce a pure amnesia with short term memory loss and the usual retrograde and antegrade components. Prognosis is reasonable provided the other hippocampus is intact, but maximum improvement may take up to three months. Some events in the basilar distribution produce amnesia associated with florid confabulation and sleep disturbance. Sometimes a variety of visual disturbances are associated, such as cortical blindness, visual disorientation, field defect, and defects of gaze (often upwards). Amnesia with visual defects occurs after resuscitation from cardiac arrest or bypass surgery. This condition, variously known as borderzone or watershed ischaemia, refers to the fringes of the basilar circulation, and has a variable prognosis; there is no treatment. Temporary amnesia may follow vertebral angiography. Any established lesion should be assessed by computed tomography so that prognosis can be given.

Multiple cerebral infarction can lead to dementia. The syndrome is unpredictable, but it can usually be distinguished from Alzheimer type dementia by the stepwise deterioration, often with relative preservation of insight and personality. Lability of mood and pseudobulbar features are pointers, as are sudden onset pyramidal tract or parietal features. The commonest cause is hypertension, but any vascular disease affecting the left heart, aorta, or carotid vessels may be a cause. The treatment is the identification and removal of the cause; it is not enough to hope that patients will not have recurrent cerebrovascular events. The most effective prevention is good antihypertensive treatment, avoidance of smoking, and early surgery in unstable carotid atheroma.

Depression

Mild depression may present with memory loss, and severe depression in the elderly may masquerade as dementia. The problem is that poor memory and concentration may be more obvious than the abnormal mood, depressive thought content, and sleep disorder. The depressed patient tends to be uninterested and inattentive but does not confabulate. Up to 10% of elderly patients thought to have dementia may make an excellent recovery with antidepressant treatment. Such opportunity must not be missed, and the presence of some cortical atrophy on tomography should not preclude a trial of such treatment.

Some patients with early or established dementia are depressed. Insight disappears early in Alzheimer's disease but may be preserved in multi-infarct dementia. Some patients with multi-infarct dementia recover much of their intellectual function when given an antidepressant.

Cerebral tumour

Rapid progression of focal signs, the onset of epilepsy, and papilloedema support the diagnosis of cerebral tumour. Slowly growing and suitably sited tumours may cause slowly progressive dementia, but headache is almost invariably present. Rarely a pure amnesic syndrome is seen in primary or secondary cerebral malignancy. Pure amnesia can develop as a non-metastatic manifestation of bronchial carcinoma, in association with encephalitic features in the cerebrospinal fluid. Tumour is diagnosed from focal electroencephalographic features, computed tomography, and angiography.

Pseudotumour cerebri

Amnesia or pseudodementia is rarely seen in pseudotumour cerebri (or benign intracranial hypertension), a diagnosis made when serious causes of raised intracranial pressure have been excluded. There are many causes, but most patients are young women. When headache is severe and amnesia present a shunt will generally be required to allow some of the excessive cerebrospinal fluid to drain into a jugular vein or the peritoneal cavity. Prognosis is excellent.

Subdural haematoma

Half of the patients with chronic subdural haematoma do not recall the injury, which may have been mild. Headache and mental change (including amnesia) are the usual complaints but both may be missed when there is confusion. Focal signs and epilepsy are pointers. Very gradual tentorial herniation can lead to unobtrusive features such as minimal ptosis and paresis of upward gaze. Subdural haematoma is diagnosed by computed tomography, may be bilateral, and should be considered in alcoholics and epileptics. Chronic subdural haematoma causing pressure symptoms requires urgent surgery.

Boxer's dementia

The tragic syndrome of dementia with ataxia, dysarthria, and parkinsonian features is rare but is a compelling argument against boxing. There is speculation that forms of dancing involving violent head movement may have the same long term result.

Occult hydrocephalus

Though rare, occult hydrocephalus is important because early treatment produces good results. The clue is the history of meningitis, intracranial haemorrhage, or head injury. The features are dementia with a very early amnesia, incontinence, and apraxia of gait. This is a slow, unstable, wide based, fixed footed gait with correction so poor that falling is common. There may be no motor or sensory features on examining the legs.

Neurosyphilis

Although rare, neurosyphilis has a good prognosis if treated early. The common presentation is simple dementia, not the florid grandiose confabulation that is so well known. The early features may be irritability and personality change as in some cerebral tumours. Headache is not unusual. As amnesia is often late, the differential diagnosis is from other causes of personality deterioration. Quite often there are Argyll-Robertson pupils. Diagnosis is made by examining blood or cerebrospinal fluid. Positive haemagglutination and fluorescent antibody test results in blood do not confirm active disease, but in cerebrospinal fluid a positive Veneral Diseases Research Laboratory test and raised protein concentration and lymphocytosis are confirmatory. Treatment is with penicillin, initially under corticosteroid cover.

Disorders of movement

The early signs of Huntington's chorea are irritability and anxiety-depression, with amnesia and choreiform movement later. Most patients retain insight for some time. In both Parkinson's

Memory Loss

disease and Wilson's disease intellectual deterioration is late and the underlying disease will not be suspected because of amnesia. The dementia of advanced Parkinson's disease, although sometimes an indication of cerebral disease, can be related to drug treatment, especially excessive levodopa.

General medical disorders

Hypothyroidism, vitamin B_{12} deficiency, and hypercalcaemia may all present as dementia with prominent amnesic features and in the absence of other more usual symptoms. Routine screening in dementia should always include estimation of thyroid stimulating hormone, mean cell volume, and serum calcium concentration.

Drug treatment

A full drug history must be obtained in every patient who has memory defect. Chronic dependence on sedatives, benzodiazepines, or phenothiazines and certain anticonvulsants may lead to a chronic pseudodementia in which memory failure is prominent. Digoxin and corticosteroids are less well known causes. Sulphonylureas and insulin, while they may obviously cause acute hypoglycaemia, can more unobtrusively lead to chronic hypoglycaemia, to which the patient becomes partly acclimatised. The pseudodementia usually recovers when the cause is removed; a few patients possibly sustain permanent intellectual impairment.

A wide variety of drugs cause toxic confusional states, either alone or with other causes. The list includes sedatives, anticonvulsants, antidepressants, antiparkinsonian medication, antihistamines, corticosteroids, digoxin, atropine, opiates, cycloserine, isoniazid, hypoglycaemics, and hypotensive agents. The treatment consists of reducing or withdrawing the offending drug, replacing it if necessary, correcting other contributory factors, and giving chlormethiazole or haloperidol to control overactivity or other florid features.

In younger patients solvent abuse can produce an apathetic pseudodementia. The florid hallucination of the bad lysergic acid trip is well known in casualty departments.

Toxic and metabolic confusional syndrome

In the older age group the responsibility is to identify the underlying disease in confusional syndromes, commonly chest or urine infection, myocardial infarction, or cerebral infarction. Gen-erally the treatment is that of the cause, but with medication to control the more florid manifestations. Sedatives should be avoided in chronic lung disease, severe heart failure, and acute intermittent porphyria, where the disease may be intensified. Cranial arteritis is not easy to diagnose; if suspected corticosteroid treatment should be urgently considered. Drugs are an important cause.

Encephalitic illnesses of any severity produce striking memory impairment although mingled with other features. The recovery may not be complete and the antegrade amnesia may persist longer than after head injury, and with a deeper retrograde amnesia.

Alzheimer's disease

Alzheimer's disease is responsible for up to 80% of cases of dementia. Cases occurring in people aged under 65 are described as presenile. There may be early insight, with some anxiety or depression, but this shortly disappears. A poor and deteriorating memory may be the presenting problem. The other main features are deterioration of intellect, personality and behaviour change, and focal neurological symptoms or signs. These include subtle dysphasic errors, along with apraxia and agnosia, which are recognised from an inability to dress, find the way around a familiar environment, or carry out simple tasks with everyday objects. Focal and major epilepsy is seen later in the illness along with primitive reflexes such as sucking and tonic grasp and parkinsonian features. The progress is inexorable, and death is from inanition and pneumonia.

The diagnosis is strongly suggested by dementia associated with mild organic signs but with no evidence of intracranial pressure increase or headache. Computed tomography confirms diffuse cerebral atrophy with ventricular enlargement, and brain biopsy (seldom carried out) shows fibrillary tangles and granulovacuolar degeneration. Despite biochemical evidence of certain deficiencies in the brain, there is no treatment.

Benign forgetfulness

This is the "condition" in which many middle aged and older patients are inclined to forget the names of persons or places—often temporarily. Mood and affect are normal, and formal tests of memory, intellect, and personality show nothing abnormal. Fatigue and worry may contribute. This condition is not a precursor of Alzheimer's disease and may be the commonest " amnesia" presenting to the medical profession. Reassurance is required.

WEAKNESS

KENNETH C McHARDY

The algorithm presents a diagnostic approach to patients presenting with, or found to have, some form of weakness. The main diagnostic patterns considered relate to generalised weakness and to both symmetrical and asymmetrical non-generalised weakness, though many causes of symmetrical weakness can also present in an asymmetrical manner. By its very nature an algorithm gives relatively stark information and permits little scope for considering the mode of presentation and history, both of which may give important pointers to diagnosis. Most of the diagnostic suggestions are indications for referral to a specialist.

Patients often include generalised weakness among their presenting symptoms. Generalised weakness is often due to underlying systemic disease or a neurotic or depressive problem and has a more specific neurological cause only in rare cases. When weakness is not generalised the pattern of disability is of great diagnostic importance. Hemiparesis is a familiar presentation and is usually, but by no means always, due to cerebrovascular disease. Alternative causes should be sought in younger patients and those with atypical features. Certain neurological disorders, such as multiple sclerosis or motor neurone disease, show patterns that evolve gradually, and the diagnosis may therefore not be apparent at the time of initial presentation When dealing with weakness in the legs clinicians should always consider the possibility of cord compression as immediate myelography and subsequent laminectomy can potentially prevent paraplegia. Fully developed subacute combined degeneration of the cord is only rarely seen, and clinicians should be critical of accepting this diagnosis rather than arranging myelography. Though much rarer than in the past, neurosyphilis still occasionally develops, and many would still consider serological screening to be a worthwhile routine investigation in patients with neurological complaints, par-ticularly as the meningovascular form may respond dramatically to treatment with penicillin.

The problem often arises of distinguishing between an organic and a neurotic basis for a particular patient's complaint of weakness. This may be extremely difficult, and, though certain features can be helpful, none should be regarded as foolproof. Patients with neurosis often show inconsistencies in their weakness, being unable, for example, to move a leg while under examination yet walking quite normally when less closely observed. Inconsistencies may also appear in the history if, for example, a patient has a paralysed arm but no difficulty in wearing lace-up shoes. A patient with neurosis is also more likely to have a sharply demarcated region of motor and sensory failure that is anatomically incompatible with an organic neurological lesion. There may be lack of genuine effort in complying with tests of power, often accompanied by tensing of muscles other than those under scrutiny. It must be remembered, however, that no matter how many times a neurotic individual "cries wolf," this does not render him insusceptible to organic disease. Likewise, patients showing obvious features of hysteria may none the less have some underlying organic weakness.

Further reading

Gibberd FB, ed. Neurology. *Medicine International* 1987: 1869-2003.
Walton JN. *Brain's disease of the nervous system.* 9th ed. Oxford: Oxford Medical Publications, 1985.
Weatherall DJ, Ledingham JCG, Warrell DA, eds. *Oxford textbook of medicine.* 2nd ed. Oxford: Oxford Medical Publications, 1987.
Beck ER, Francis JL, Souhami RL. *Tutorials in differential diagnosis.* 2nd ed. London: Pitman Medical, 1982.

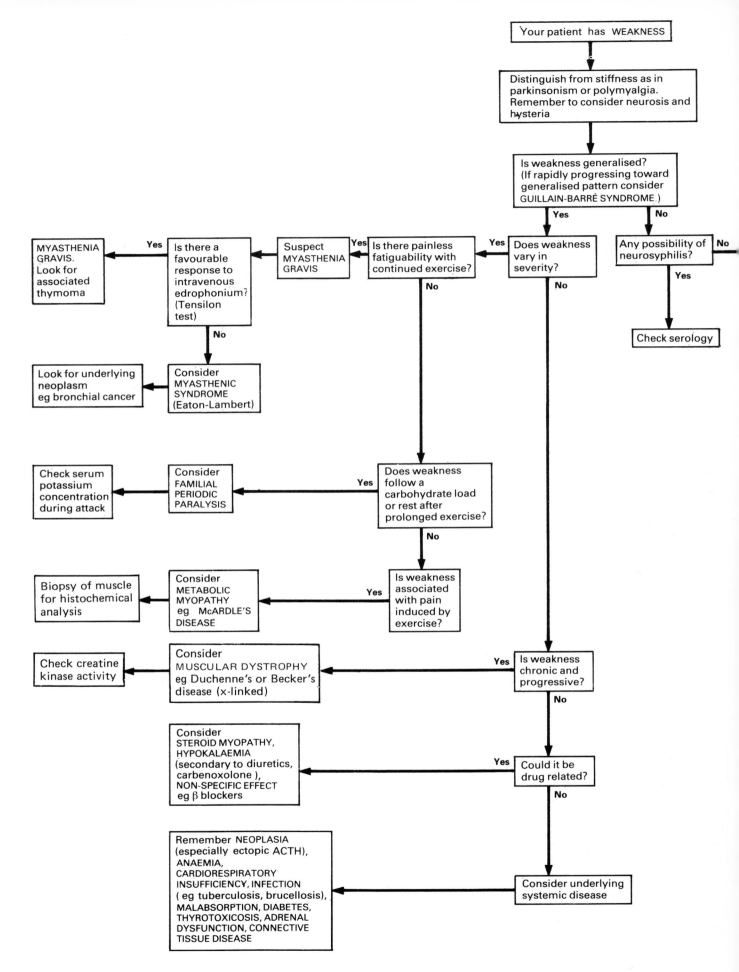

Your patient has WEAKNESS

Distinguish from stiffness as in parkinsonism or polymyalgia. Remember to consider neurosis and hysteria

Is weakness generalised? (If rapidly progressing toward generalised pattern consider GUILLAIN-BARRÉ SYNDROME.)

Yes → Does weakness vary in severity?

No → Any possibility of neurosyphilis?

No →

Yes → Check serology

Does weakness vary in severity? **Yes** → Is there painless fatiguability with continued exercise? **Yes** → Suspect MYASTHENIA GRAVIS → Is there a favourable response to intravenous edrophonium? (Tensilon test) **Yes** → MYASTHENIA GRAVIS. Look for associated thymoma

Is there a favourable response to intravenous edrophonium? **No** → Consider MYASTHENIC SYNDROME (Eaton-Lambert) → Look for underlying neoplasm eg bronchial cancer

Is there painless fatiguability with continued exercise? **No** ↓

Does weakness vary in severity? **No** ↓

Does weakness follow a carbohydrate load or rest after prolonged exercise? **Yes** → Consider FAMILIAL PERIODIC PARALYSIS → Check serum potassium concentration during attack

No ↓

Is weakness associated with pain induced by exercise? **Yes** → Consider METABOLIC MYOPATHY eg McARDLE'S DISEASE → Biopsy of muscle for histochemical analysis

Is weakness chronic and progressive? **Yes** → Consider MUSCULAR DYSTROPHY eg Duchenne's or Becker's disease (x-linked) → Check creatine kinase activity

No ↓

Could it be drug related? **Yes** → Consider STEROID MYOPATHY, HYPOKALAEMIA (secondary to diuretics, carbenoxolone), NON-SPECIFIC EFFECT eg β blockers

No ↓

Consider underlying systemic disease → Remember NEOPLASIA (especially ectopic ACTH), ANAEMIA, CARDIORESPIRATORY INSUFFICIENCY, INFECTION (eg tuberculosis, brucellosis), MALABSORPTION, DIABETES, THYROTOXICOSIS, ADRENAL DYSFUNCTION, CONNECTIVE TISSUE DISEASE

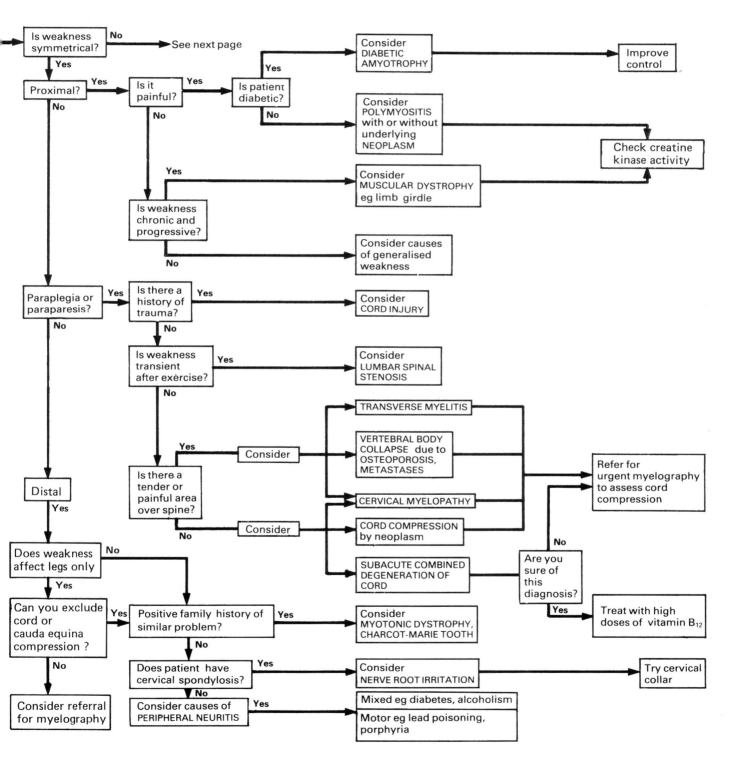

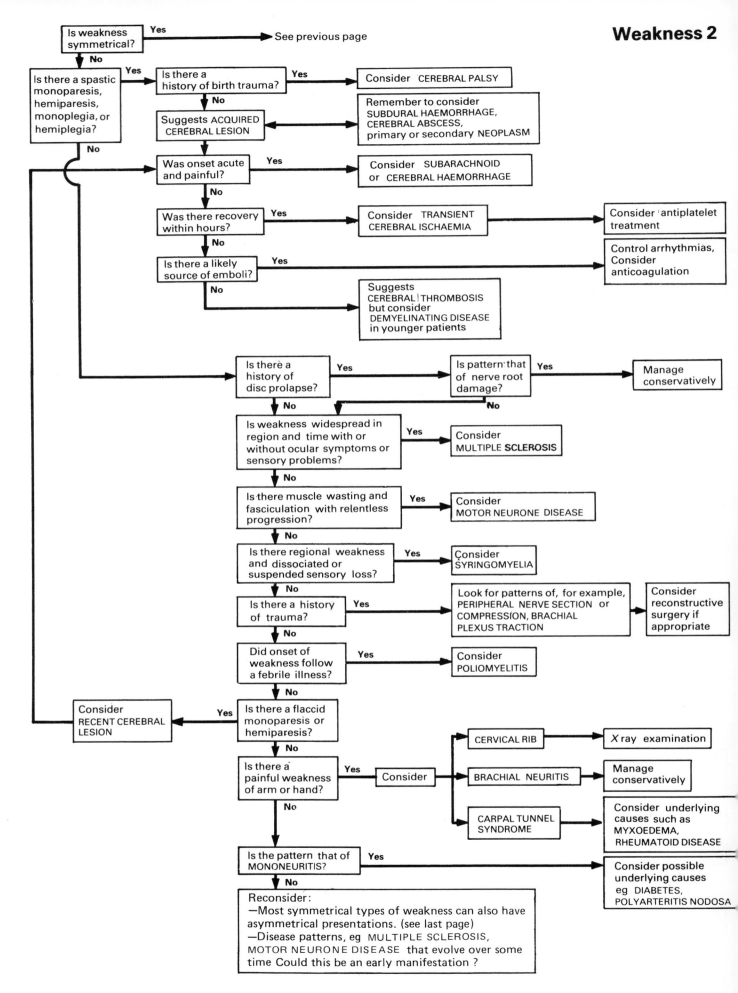

Is weakness symmetrical? — Yes → See previous page

No ↓

Is there a spastic monoparesis, hemiparesis, monoplegia, or hemiplegia?

— Yes → Is there a history of birth trauma? — Yes → Consider CEREBRAL PALSY

No ↓

Suggests ACQUIRED CEREBRAL LESION ← Remember to consider SUBDURAL HAEMORRHAGE, CEREBRAL ABSCESS, primary or secondary NEOPLASM

↓

Was onset acute and painful? — Yes → Consider SUBARACHNOID or CEREBRAL HAEMORRHAGE

No ↓

Was there recovery within hours? — Yes → Consider TRANSIENT CEREBRAL ISCHAEMIA → Consider antiplatelet treatment

No ↓

Is there a likely source of emboli? — Yes → Control arrhythmias, Consider anticoagulation

No ↓

Suggests CEREBRAL THROMBOSIS but consider DEMYELINATING DISEASE in younger patients

---

Is there a history of disc prolapse? — Yes → Is pattern that of nerve root damage? — Yes → Manage conservatively

No ↓ / No ←

Is weakness widespread in region and time with or without ocular symptoms or sensory problems? — Yes → Consider MULTIPLE SCLEROSIS

No ↓

Is there muscle wasting and fasciculation with relentless progression? — Yes → Consider MOTOR NEURONE DISEASE

No ↓

Is there regional weakness and dissociated or suspended sensory loss? — Yes → Consider SYRINGOMYELIA

No ↓

Is there a history of trauma? — Yes → Look for patterns of, for example, PERIPHERAL NERVE SECTION or COMPRESSION, BRACHIAL PLEXUS TRACTION → Consider reconstructive surgery if appropriate

No ↓

Did onset of weakness follow a febrile illness? — Yes → Consider POLIOMYELITIS

No ↓

Is there a flaccid monoparesis or hemiparesis? — Yes → Consider RECENT CEREBRAL LESION

No ↓

Is there a painful weakness of arm or hand? — Yes → Consider:
- CERVICAL RIB → X ray examination
- BRACHIAL NEURITIS → Manage conservatively
- CARPAL TUNNEL SYNDROME → Consider underlying causes such as MYXOEDEMA, RHEUMATOID DISEASE

No ↓

Is the pattern that of MONONEURITIS? — Yes → Consider possible underlying causes eg DIABETES, POLYARTERITIS NODOSA

No ↓

Reconsider:
—Most symmetrical types of weakness can also have asymmetrical presentations. (see last page)
—Disease patterns, eg MULTIPLE SCLEROSIS, MOTOR NEURONE DISEASE that evolve over some time Could this be an early manifestation ?

INCOORDINATION

KENNETH C McHARDY

This algorithm addresses the problem of diagnosis in a patient whose presentation may range from unsteadiness of gait, through minor clumsiness with, for example, crockery, to a distinct inability to perform fine motor tasks smoothly and efficiently. Some possible underlying problems, such as dizziness or tremor, are dealt with elsewhere in this series. In view of the increasing prevalence of alcohol abuse, acute and chronic disorders related to alcohol consumption and presenting with incoordination are increasingly likely to be met. Drug treatment is also a potentially common cause, particularly with the vast quantities of long acting benzodiazepine hypnotics, such as nitrazepam and flurazepam, prescribed to elderly people. With its propensity to affect the cerebellum and its connections the features of multiple sclerosis should also be sought.

Finally, previously undetected myxoedema, which occasionally presents with incoordination as a major symptom, is rewarding to diagnose and treat.

Further reading

Gibberd FB, ed. Neurology. *Medicine International* 1987: 1869-2003.
Walton JN. *Brain's disease of the nervous system.* 9th ed. Oxford: Oxford Medical Publications, 1985.
Weatherall DJ, Ledingham JCG, Warrell DA, eds. *Oxford textbook of medicine.* 2nd ed. Oxford: Oxford Medical Publications, 1987.
Beck ER, Francis JL, Souhami RL. *Tutorials in differential diagnosis.* 2nd ed. London: Pitman Medical, 1982.

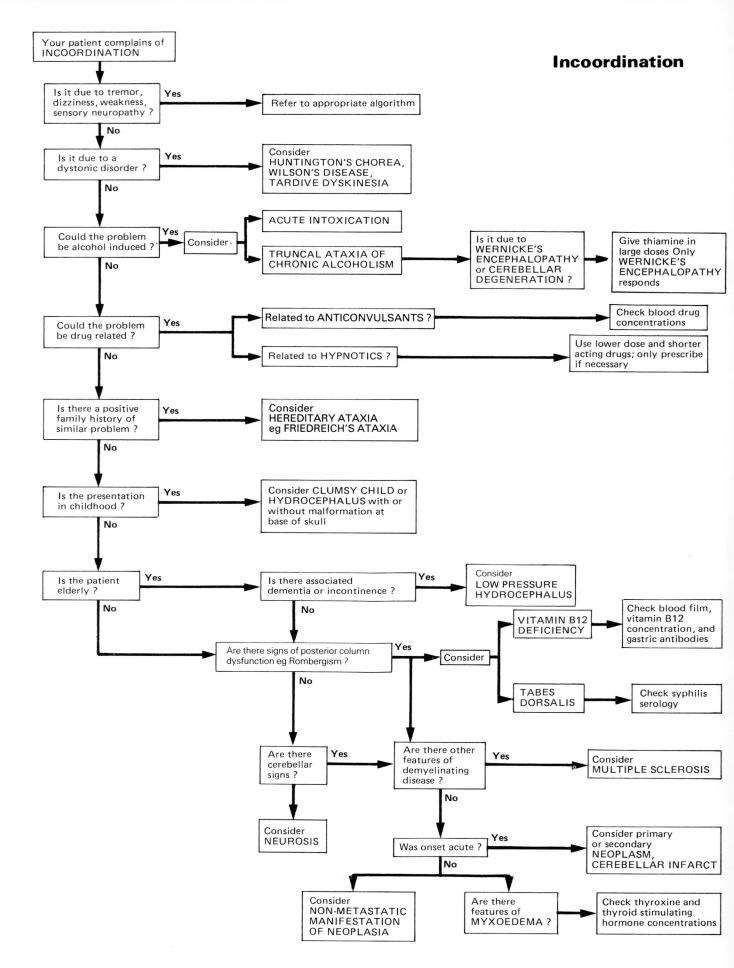

Your patient complains of INCOORDINATION

Is it due to tremor, dizziness, weakness, sensory neuropathy ? — **Yes** → Refer to appropriate algorithm

No

Is it due to a dystonic disorder ? — **Yes** → Consider HUNTINGTON'S CHOREA, WILSON'S DISEASE, TARDIVE DYSKINESIA

No

Could the problem be alcohol induced ? — **Yes** → Consider · → ACUTE INTOXICATION

TRUNCAL ATAXIA OF CHRONIC ALCOHOLISM → Is it due to WERNICKE'S ENCEPHALOPATHY or CEREBELLAR DEGENERATION ? → Give thiamine in large doses Only WERNICKE'S ENCEPHALOPATHY responds

No

Could the problem be drug related ? — **Yes** → Related to ANTICONVULSANTS ? → Check blood drug concentrations

Related to HYPNOTICS ? → Use lower dose and shorter acting drugs; only prescribe if necessary

No

Is there a positive family history of similar problem ? — **Yes** → Consider HEREDITARY ATAXIA eg FRIEDREICH'S ATAXIA

No

Is the presentation in childhood ? — **Yes** → Consider CLUMSY CHILD or HYDROCEPHALUS with or without malformation at base of skull

No

Is the patient elderly ? — **Yes** → Is there associated dementia or incontinence ? — **Yes** → Consider LOW PRESSURE HYDROCEPHALUS

No

Are there signs of posterior column dysfunction eg Rombergism ? — **Yes** → Consider → VITAMIN B12 DEFICIENCY → Check blood film, vitamin B12 concentration, and gastric antibodies

TABES DORSALIS → Check syphilis serology

No

Are there cerebellar signs ? — **Yes** → Are there other features of demyelinating disease ? — **Yes** → Consider MULTIPLE SCLEROSIS

No

Consider NEUROSIS

Was onset acute ? — **Yes** → Consider primary or secondary NEOPLASM, CEREBELLAR INFARCT

No

Consider NON-METASTATIC MANIFESTATION OF NEOPLASIA

Are there features of MYXOEDEMA ? → Check thyroxine and thyroid stimulating hormone concentrations

LOSS OF VISION

M J JAMIESON, H M A TOWLER

A common and often major handicap, visual loss may be preventable and is often symptomatic of treatable intraocular and extraocular disease. Diagnosis of its underlying cause is often possible without specialist experience or equipment. Early diagnosis by a general practitioner or general physician may lead to early treatment and will be a useful guide to prompt and appropriate referral, avoiding time consuming and perhaps unnecessary referral to opticians and ophthalmologists. In particular, chronic glaucoma may be detected early, refractive errors diagnosed and referred for retinoscopy, diabetic and hypertensive retinopathy found and appropriately managed, and disorders primarily of the central nervous system identified. This algorithm attempts to provide routes to diagnosis in cases where visual loss is the dominant symptom. Conditions in which pain predominates but where visual impairment may be present—for example, acute glaucoma, acute iritis—are discussed only briefly. Conditions that are common world wide but rare in the United Kingdom—for example, vitamin A deficiency and infective diseases such as trachoma and onchocerciasis—are not considered further.

History

The history should define the onset, progress, duration and extent of visual loss. In particular, try to distinguish between sudden *awareness* of visual loss and sudden *development* of visual loss. The distinction between central and peripheral loss is also useful. Central visual loss presents as impairment of visual acuity and implies defective retinal image formation (through refractive error or opacity in the ocular media), or macular, or optic nerve dysfunction. Peripheral field loss is more often clinically silent, particularly when the onset is gradual. It usually implies extramacular retinal disease or a defect in the visual pathway (optic nerve, chiasm, tract, radiation or cortex). There are, however, areas of overlap as the algorithm shows, and disorders may coexist.

The drug history may be relevant. Visual disorders that have been associated with drugs are listed in the table.

Examination

Examination should include measurement of visual acuity, testing of pupillary reflexes, assessment of visual fields, direct ophthalmoscopy and when possible, measurement of intraocular pressure and colour vision. Distant and near visual acuity can be assessed with Snellen Chart and British Faculty of Ophthalmologists' reading type, respectively. Detection of an afferent pupillary defect by the "swinging flashlight" test is a valuable clinical sign which usually indicates optic nerve dysfunction but which may occur with extensive retinal lesions—for example, retinal detachment—or lesions of the optic tract. A bright light is swung between the pupils every two to four seconds: normally each pupil constricts when the light is swung on to it, indicating that the direct and consensual responses are of equal magnitude. If the direct response is impaired relative to the consensual response—that is, a relative afferent defect—the

Visual disorders associated with drugs

Disorder	Drug
Corneal opacities	Amiodarone Hydroxychloroquine Chlorpromazine Vitamin D Indomethacin Chlorpropamide
Precipitation of acute narrow angle glaucoma	Mydriatic drops Tricyclics Antihistamines
Refractive changes	Thiazides
Lens opacities	Corticosteroids Phenothiazines
Retinopathy	Hydroxychloroquine Chloroquine Thioridazine (other phenothiazines less commonly) Tamoxifen
Papilloedema (24° to benign intracranial hypertension)	Oral contraceptives Corticosteroids Tetracyclines Nalidixic acid Vitamin A
Optic neuropathy	Ethanol Tobacco Ethambutol Disulfiram

pupil on the affected side will be seen to dilate when the light is swung on to it.

Confrontation testing will detect major field defects and can be refined by using smaller targets such as 5 mm hat pins, thus allowing central and paracentral scotomata to be detected. Visual inattention is best detected by confrontation and will be missed by formal perimetry.

Before examining the fundus look for the red reflex at the pupil. Small opacities in the ocular media such as early cataract or vitreous condensations ("floaters") appear black against the red background. Larger opacities may obscure the reflex entirely.

A short acting mydriatic, such as tropicamide, should be used to dilate the pupils before fundoscopy. The macula and retinal periphery can only be satisfactorily examined through a dilated pupil. The risk of precipitating acute narrow angle glaucoma is low, but caution should be exercised, particularly in long-sighted patients. Simple examination of the spectacles will differentiate long and short sightedness: a long sighted person's spectacles magnify; spectacles for short sightedness reduce size of the image. Patients should be instructed to report back if the eye becomes painful.

Intraocular pressure cannot be reliably assessed by digital examination, unless very high.

Acquired red-green colour defects can be detected with Ishihara pseudoisochromatic colour plates which are therefore useful in detecting optic nerve dysfunction early and in assessing its progress.

The pinhole test is useful if refractive error is suspected. A 1 mm pinhole will correct about ± 5 dioptres of refractive error, though some improvement may also be seen with corneal or lens opacities. The pinhole will not improve visual acuity, or may worsen it, in macular or optic nerve lesions.

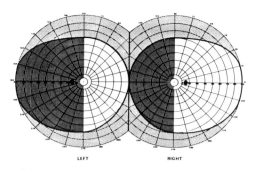

Left homonymous hemianopia
sparing macula

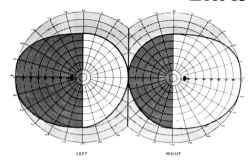

Left homonymous hemianopia
splitting macula

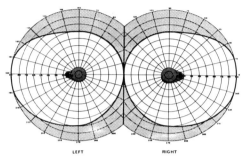

Bilateral centrocaecal
(ie involving the blind
spot) scotomas, eg toxic
optic neuropathy following
methanol ingestion

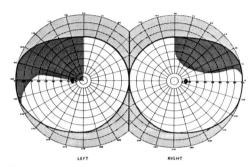

Upper bitemporal
quadrantanopia due to
a pituitary adenoma

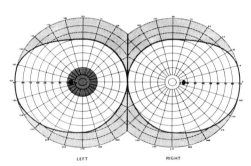

Left central scotoma, eg optic
neuritis or senile macular
degeneration

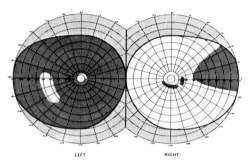

Glaucomatous field loss. Constricted left
field with nasal step and temporal island
of vision. Inferior arcuate scotomas and
temporal wedge defect in the right
field

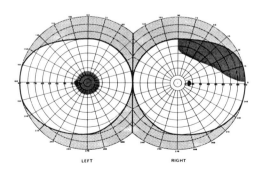

Left central scotoma plus right
superotemporal ("junctional")
defect respecting the vertical
meridian indicating a lesion
involving the anterior optic
chiasm

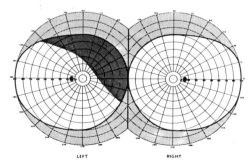

Superonasal left field loss crossing
the vertical and horizontal meridia
due to an intraocular lesion, e.g.
retinal detachment

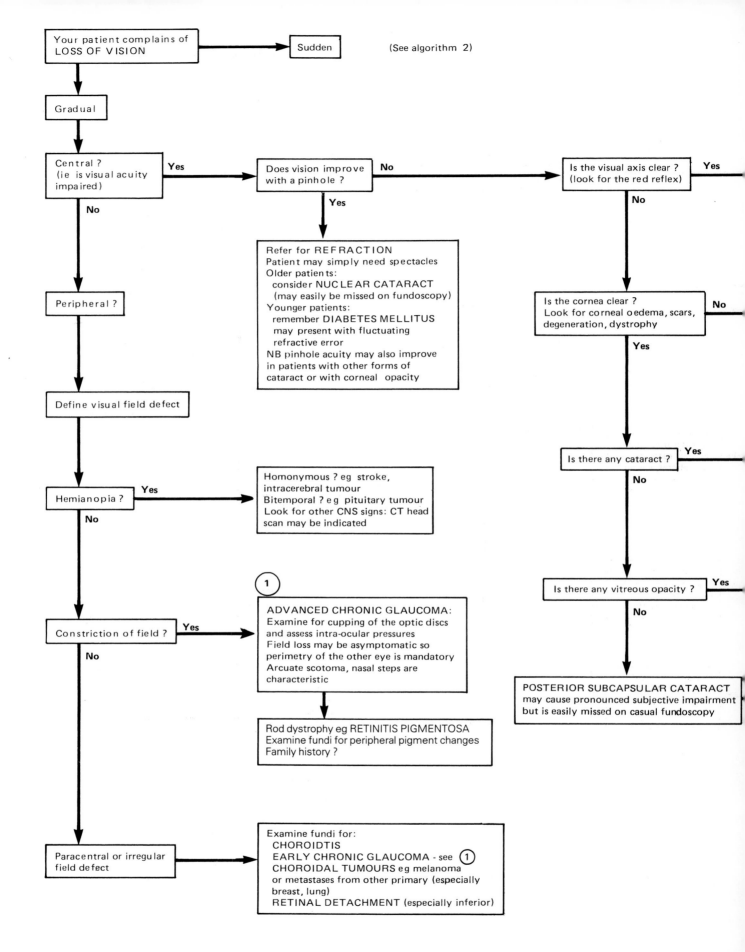

Your patient complains of
LOSS OF VISION

→ Sudden   (See algorithm 2)

Gradual

Central ?
(ie is visual acuity
impaired)

Yes → Does vision improve
with a pinhole ?

No → Is the visual axis clear ?
(look for the red reflex) **Yes**

Yes ↓

Refer for REFRACTION
Patient may simply need spectacles
Older patients:
  consider NUCLEAR CATARACT
  (may easily be missed on fundoscopy)
Younger patients:
  remember DIABETES MELLITUS
  may present with fluctuating
  refractive error
NB pinhole acuity may also improve
in patients with other forms of
cataract or with corneal opacity

No ↓

Is the cornea clear ?
Look for corneal oedema, scars,
degeneration, dystrophy **No**

Yes ↓

Peripheral ?

Define visual field defect

Is there any cataract ? **Yes**

No ↓

Hemianopia ?   **Yes** →

Homonymous ? eg stroke,
intracerebral tumour
Bitemporal ? eg pituitary tumour
Look for other CNS signs: CT head
scan may be indicated

No

Is there any vitreous opacity ? **Yes**

No ↓

① ADVANCED CHRONIC GLAUCOMA:
Examine for cupping of the optic discs
and assess intra-ocular pressures
Field loss may be asymptomatic so
perimetry of the other eye is mandatory
Arcuate scotoma, nasal steps are
characteristic

Constriction of field ? **Yes** →

No

Rod dystrophy eg RETINITIS PIGMENTOSA
Examine fundi for peripheral pigment changes
Family history ?

POSTERIOR SUBCAPSULAR CATARACT
may cause pronounced subjective impairment
but is easily missed on casual fundoscopy

Paracentral or irregular
field defect →

Examine fundi for:
  CHOROIDTIS
  EARLY CHRONIC GLAUCOMA - see ①
  CHOROIDAL TUMOURS eg melanoma
  or metastases from other primary (especially
  breast, lung)
  RETINAL DETACHMENT (especially inferior)

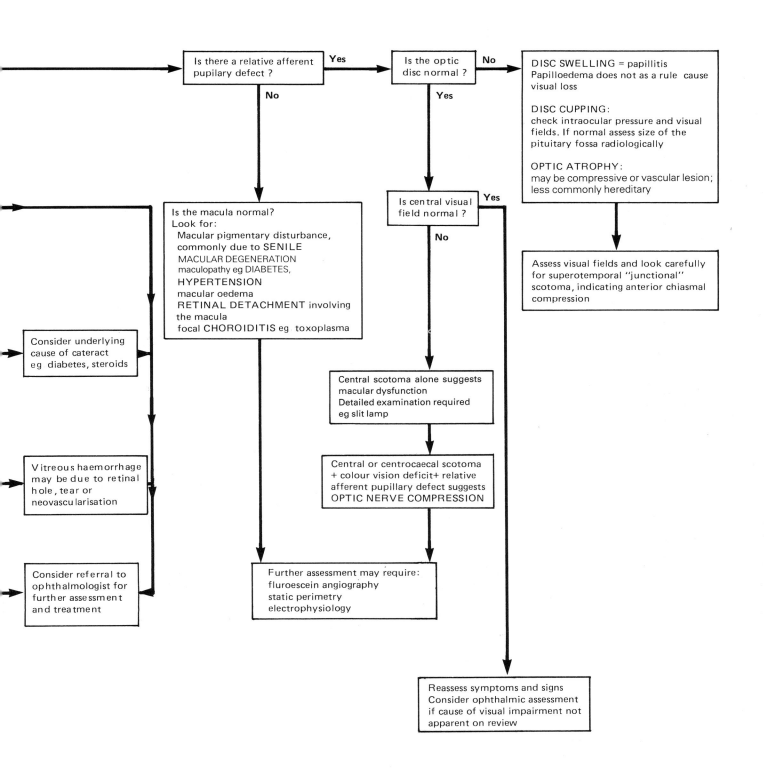

Is there a relative afferent pupilary defect ?

Yes → Is the optic disc normal ?

No →
DISC SWELLING = papillitis
Papilloedema does not as a rule cause visual loss

DISC CUPPING:
check intraocular pressure and visual fields. If normal assess size of the pituitary fossa radiologically

OPTIC ATROPHY:
may be compressive or vascular lesion; less commonly hereditary

No →

Is the macula normal?
Look for:
Macular pigmentary disturbance, commonly due to SENILE
MACULAR DEGENERATION
maculopathy eg DIABETES,
HYPERTENSION
macular oedema
RETINAL DETACHMENT involving the macula
focal CHOROIDITIS eg toxoplasma

Yes (disc normal) →

Is central visual field normal ?

Yes →

Assess visual fields and look carefully for superotemporal "junctional" scotoma, indicating anterior chiasmal compression

No →

Central scotoma alone suggests macular dysfunction
Detailed examination required eg slit lamp

Central or centrocaecal scotoma
+ colour vision deficit+ relative afferent pupillary defect suggests
OPTIC NERVE COMPRESSION

Consider underlying cause of cateract eg diabetes, steroids

Vitreous haemorrhage may be due to retinal hole, tear or neovascularisation

Consider referral to ophthalmologist for further assessment and treatment

Further assessment may require:
fluroescein angiography
static perimetry
electrophysiology

Reassess symptoms and signs
Consider ophthalmic assessment if cause of visual impairment not apparent on review

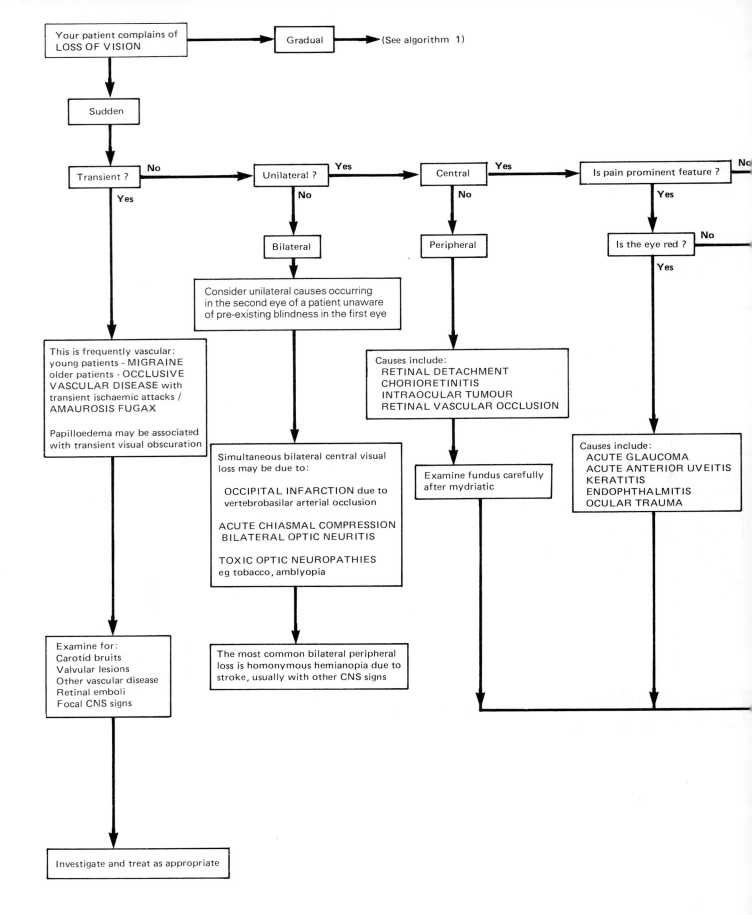

Your patient complains of LOSS OF VISION → Gradual → (See algorithm 1)

Sudden

Transient ? — No → Unilateral ? — Yes → Central — Yes → Is pain prominent feature ? — No

Transient ? — Yes

Unilateral ? — No → Bilateral

Central — No → Peripheral

Is pain prominent feature ? — Yes → Is the eye red ? — No

Is the eye red ? — Yes

This is frequently vascular:
young patients - MIGRAINE
older patients - OCCLUSIVE
VASCULAR DISEASE with
transient ischaemic attacks /
AMAUROSIS FUGAX

Papilloedema may be associated
with transient visual obscuration

Consider unilateral causes occurring
in the second eye of a patient unaware
of pre-existing blindness in the first eye

Causes include:
RETINAL DETACHMENT
CHORIORETINITIS
INTRAOCULAR TUMOUR
RETINAL VASCULAR OCCLUSION

Simultaneous bilateral central visual
loss may be due to:

OCCIPITAL INFARCTION due to
vertebrobasilar arterial occlusion

ACUTE CHIASMAL COMPRESSION
BILATERAL OPTIC NEURITIS

TOXIC OPTIC NEUROPATHIES
eg tobacco, amblyopia

Examine fundus carefully
after mydriatic

Causes include:
ACUTE GLAUCOMA
ACUTE ANTERIOR UVEITIS
KERATITIS
ENDOPHTHALMITIS
OCULAR TRAUMA

Examine for:
Carotid bruits
Valvular lesions
Other vascular disease
Retinal emboli
Focal CNS signs

The most common bilateral peripheral
loss is homonymous hemianopia due to
stroke, usually with other CNS signs

Investigate and treat as appropriate

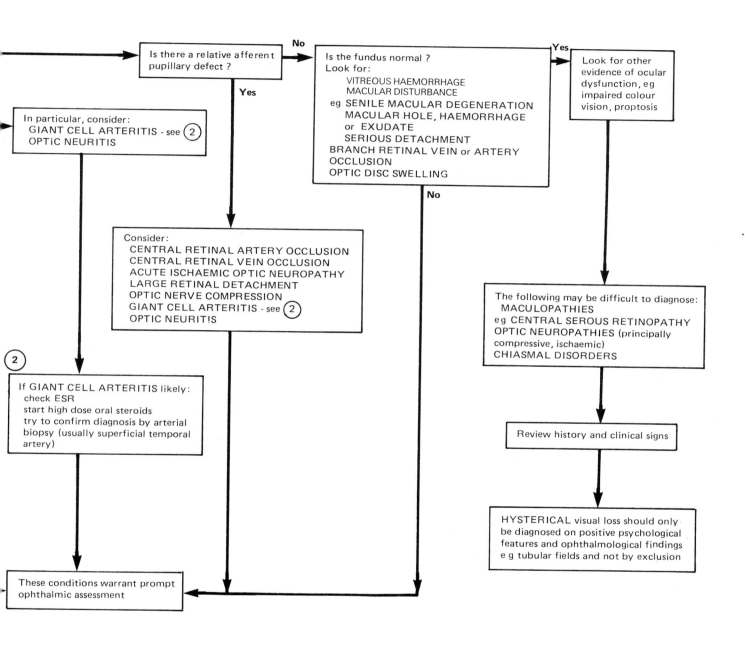

Is there a relative afferent pupillary defect ?

No → Is the fundus normal ?
Look for:
    VITREOUS HAEMORRHAGE
    MACULAR DISTURBANCE
eg SENILE MACULAR DEGENERATION
    MACULAR HOLE, HAEMORRHAGE
    or EXUDATE
    SERIOUS DETACHMENT
BRANCH RETINAL VEIN or ARTERY
OCCLUSION
OPTIC DISC SWELLING

Yes → Look for other evidence of ocular dysfunction, eg impaired colour vision, proptosis

In particular, consider:
GIANT CELL ARTERITIS - see ②
OPTIC NEURITIS

Yes ↓ Consider:
CENTRAL RETINAL ARTERY OCCLUSION
CENTRAL RETINAL VEIN OCCLUSION
ACUTE ISCHAEMIC OPTIC NEUROPATHY
LARGE RETINAL DETACHMENT
OPTIC NERVE COMPRESSION
GIANT CELL ARTERITIS - see ②
OPTIC NEURITIS

No ↓

The following may be difficult to diagnose:
MACULOPATHIES
eg CENTRAL SEROUS RETINOPATHY
OPTIC NEUROPATHIES (principally compressive, ischaemic)
CHIASMAL DISORDERS

② If GIANT CELL ARTERITIS likely:
check ESR
start high dose oral steroids
try to confirm diagnosis by arterial biopsy (usually superficial temporal artery)

Review history and clinical signs

HYSTERICAL visual loss should only be diagnosed on positive psychological features and ophthalmological findings e g tubular fields and not by exclusion

These conditions warrant prompt ophthalmic assessment

Loss of Vision

Management

Opportunities for management by non-specialists are limited and most patients will need appropriate referral. Visual upset may result from systemic disease; for example, retinal vein occlusion may be the presenting symptom of hypertension or diabetes.

Vision may occasionally be restored after central retinal artery occlusion if effective treatment is given within three or four hours of onset and especially if the occlusion is embolic. The patient should lie flat and the attempted lowering of intraocular pressure should be made by brief, intermittent massage of the globe. Using both index fingers, apply firm pressure—ask the patient to look down for about 20 seconds—and repeat this after an interval. More prolonged compression may increase intraocular pressure and further impair retinal perfusion.

Giant cell arteritis should always be borne in mind as a cause of visual loss in the elderly, in whom typical systemic symptoms may not be apparent. If the diagnosis is suspected start high dose steroids (minimum 60 mg prednisolone a day initially) and arrange for arterial biopsy. The principal aim of treatment is to prevent blindness in the other eye as the presenting eye is usually severely visually impaired with little prospect of recovery. Patients should be warned to report immediately should any symptoms develop in the "good" eye. Unfortunately, many patients present late, when vision is impaired in the second eye.

Index